TYPE 2 DIABETIC COOKBOOK AND MEAL PLAN

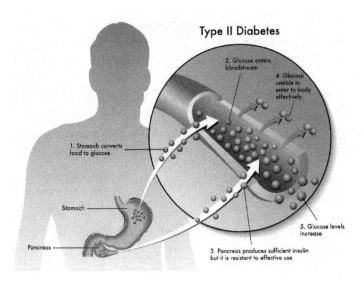

information is without contract or any type of guarantee assurance.

The trademarks that are used are without any consent and the publication of the trademark is without permission or backing by the trademark owner. All trademarks and brands within this book are for clarifying purposes only and are the owned by the owners themselves, not affiliated with this document

ABOUT THE BOOK

When it comes to diabetes, vigilance can not only eliminate the need of insulin but can also help you control your diabetes. Most people with type II diabetes, often don't attempt to control their condition. So by you following the proper diet, people with type II in diabetes, would have to prolong the need of insulin or will have to use more convenient medication to treat their condition.

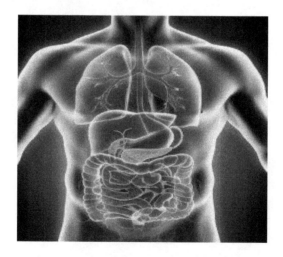

The main problem of people with diabetes is the breaking down of carbohydrates in the system. In order to have a balanced diet, unique carbohydrates in your body include anything to do with rich white flour, so as to avoid sugar. Carbohydrates include some vegetables, fruits, potatoes and white bread pasta. The different effects to the blood stream is the contribution of carbohydrates. And since diabetic people have a difficult time when breaking down any carbohydrates in their blood system those people with the highest glycemic index rating a highly likely to take the longest time when breaking down the bloodstream and a most likely to cause harm.

When following a diet plan which limits the amount of carbohydrates, you should make sure you are highly aware of the glycemic index. And try to make sure you find the right amount of good carbohydrates that are less harmful to a diabetic diet, since this is a highly threatening condition. If you have just found out that you have been diagnosed with a diabetes and the doctor has not recommended anything yet, then following the instructions and stop that practice that continues to remain the most non compliant and tend to be more denial than any other group of patients. So you can leave the full normal lifespan by following a good diabetes diet and by taking your medication.

The fact that many people are continuing to to be diagnosed with diabetes is very unfortunate. But it is good news that you can find lots of cookbooks in the market today on diabetic diet which can help a person with this condition. It takes some time for diabetic to take its toll in a human body. So you should make sure that you follow a good diabetic diet to reduce the toll of the disease and live fruitful life.

To avoid complications that may arise from this disease, it is very important to be aware of the gylcemic index, see your doctor regularly, keep up to date with the your diabetic diet, monitor your blood sugar level and make sure you take your medications as prescribed always.

By the way, upon first being diagnosed with diabetes, many patients ask can a good diet keep diabetes at bay. Most doctors will agree that a good diet, low in carbohydrates and sugars can help a person with diabetes avoid many of the complications that often accompany the disease. While a good diet can not necessarily cure the illness, a good diet can keep diabetes at bay.

Table of Contents

INTRODUCTION
TYPE 2 DIABETES

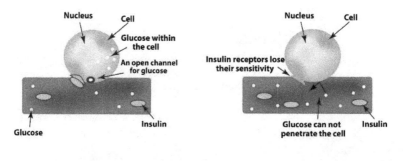

NORMAL   TYPE 2 DIABETES

Diabetes has become an alarming disease. It has reached epidemic proportions in the United States. It is time for the general public to be conscious about it. For people with diabetes, extra care in picking their diet will not only let them control the disease, it can also help them do away with insulin. Doctors often prescribe pills or tablets for most diabetics in an effort to stabilize their condition before resorting to any use of insulin. Choosing a diet specially programmed for people with diabetes can help them prolong the treatment of their ailment with medication and thereby postpone the use of insulin.

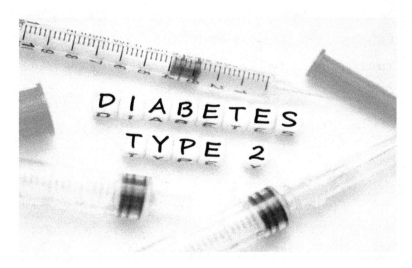

People who suffer from diabetes have problems breaking down and assimilating carbohydrates into their system.

Carbohydrates are a fairly big group or cluster of foods that people need for a balanced diet. Sugar, which many people think diabetics must stay away from, is only one example or component of carbohydrates. Aside from white sugar, other elements of carbohydrates can be found in pasta, white bread, some vegetables, potatoes, fruits, and any food with high content of white flour.

Carbohydrates constitute a complex assemblage of foods. Different groups give rise to different conditions in the blood stream. Although people with diabetes have problems breaking down carbohydrates in general, the most difficult process happens with carbohydrates that rate high in the Glycemic Index. Foods with the highest Glycemic Index rating also pose the greatest harm for diabetics.

A diet for people with diabetes allows them to limit their intake of harmful carbohydrates as indicated in the Glycemic Index. Those who have been diagnosed with Type 2 diabetes, and given medication as well as diet suggestions by their doctors, would do very well to heed the doctors' advice. Studies show that people with diabetes tend to be more in denial and non-compliant compared to other categories of patients. This should not be the case. By electing to follow rigorously a diet for people with diabetes and taking the prescribed medication, diabetics can still live to the fullest.

A diet for people with diabetes is low in carbohydrates and high in protein. Sugars and white flour must be discarded. Rice, pasta and any food that is rich in carbohydrates, should be avoided. The low carbohydrate diet that was fashionable years ago can be helpful for diabetics. Such a diet had at varying degrees very limited content of carbohydrates. Also helpful are diabetic cookbooks which diabetics can use to prepare a diet that effectively responds to their needs.

The bad news is many people continue to be found having diabetes. The good news is there is now a growing body of information about cookbooks and diets for people with diabetes that is available in the market or through the internet. Diabetes puts a heavy strain on the human body. Having a healthy diet can reduce the ill-effects of the disease on the body and allow diabetics to live a fruitful and longer lives.

It is important for diabetics to get themselves familiar with the Glycemic Index, rigorously follow a diet prescribed for people with diabetes, get their blood sugar levels regularly monitored and take their medication per doctor's prescription. This is the only way they can keep their disease in check and prevent many of its dreaded complications from arising.

TYPE 2 DIABETES MEAL PLAN

it's possible to eat deliciously with diabetes-especially in the summer when fruits and vegetables are ripe and in season. If you're feeling overwhelmed by the idea of planning your meals, try following a meal plan for a few days to see what a healthy eating plan should look like.

What makes this a healthy meal plan for diabetes?

We've included whole-grain carbohydrates to help keep you satisfied.

We cut back on saturated fats and sodium, which may negatively impact health.

The carbohydrates are balanced throughout the day with a goal of 3-4 carb servings (45-60 grams of carbohydrates) at each meal.

Each snack contains about 1 carb serving (15 grams of carbohydrates).

We've even saved room for dessert and drinks so you have healthy options when you have a craving.

How many daily calories should you aim for? Talk to your doctor or dietitian to determine what's right for you based on your age, activity level and weight-loss goals. In this plan, the calorie and carbohydrate totals are listed next to each meal and snack so you can swap in foods with similar nutrition as you like. And don't forget about leftovers! Save yourself some time by trading a lunch recipe for last night's dinner. Mix up your routine with these easy and delicious recipes that will have you out of the kitchen-and enjoying all that summer has to offer.

STOMACH PROBLEMS DUE TO DIABETES EXPLAINED

As a diabetic you are probably aware that you are at risk of suffering one or more of the awful health problems this disease can cause... heart disease... stroke... kidney disease... nerve damage... neuropathy of the feet and hands... and damaged eyes due to glaucoma, cataracts and retinopathy.

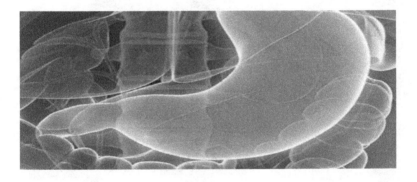

You can also end up with severe stomach problems. Here's why:

The vagus nerve controls the muscles of the stomach and intestines. This nerve, like the other nerves in your body, can be damaged if you fail to control your blood glucose levels. This condition is called gastroparesis.

When the vagus nerve is damaged, the flow of food through your stomach is interrupted, your digestion slows down, and food remains in your body for much longer than it should. Indeed, the length of time your food takes to be digested becomes unpredictable.

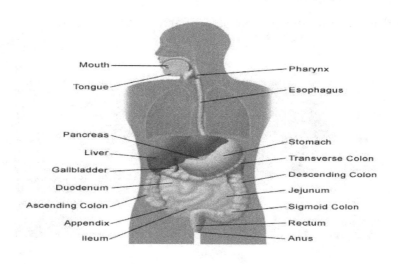

Consequences of gastroparesis

This makes it very difficult to monitor your blood glucose and effectively control the effects diabetes is having on your heart, kidneys, nerves, feet and hands, and eyes.

Gastroparesis often has further extremely unpleasant consequences:

Food stays in your stomach for too long so it spoils and you end up with a bacterial infection.

Undigested food can harden and form a lump (called a bezoar) that blocks your stomach and prevents your food moving into the small intestine.

Your stomach acids backup into your oesophagus and damage your throat, a condition known as acid reflux.

You experience nausea and vomiting. In severe cases, vomiting can leave you dehydrated.

You could feel full quickly when eating and experience abdominal bloating.

You could suffer from malnutrition, weight loss and sever fatigue due to vomiting and/or poor appetite.

Though gastroparesis is more common in persons with type 1 diabetes, persons with type 2 can also suffer from it.

Gastroparesis usually only develops after years of high blood glucose levels. In fact, most type 2 diabetics with gastroparesis will have been diabetic for at least 10 years and have been failing to control their blood glucose levels. As a consequence, they are also likely to have some of the other health problems associated with diabetes.

The best thing you can do is to prevent gastroparesis in the first place... by gaining control of your blood glucose levels before the condition starts developing.

HOW IS GASTROPARESIS DIAGNOSED?

Once your symptoms suggest that you may have gastroparesis, there are various tests that can be performed to confirm a diagnosis. These include tests that employ:

Radioactive substances:

Barium x-ray... you drink a liquid containing barium (aka a barium swallow) which coats your oesophagus, stomach and small intestine and shows up on an x-ray which can be interpreted for gastroparesis.

Barium meal... you eat a meal with barium in it. A series of x-rays will show how long it takes to digest your meal, ie how quickly your stomach empties. Too slow and you have gastroparesis.

Radioisotope gastric-emptying scan... you eat food containing a radioactive substance. If a scan shows that more than half your meal is still in your stomach after one-and-a-half hours then you have gastroparesis.

Intrusive methods:

Gastric manometry... a thin tube is inserted into your stomach through your mouth and throat to measure how quickly your food is digested.

Wireless motility capsule... is a tiny device that you swallow with a meal. Motility describes the contraction of the muscles that propel food through your gastrointestinal tract. The capsule measures the pressure, temperature and acidity of different parts in your gut and sends this data in the form of radio signals.

Upper endoscopy... in which an endoscope (thin tube) is passed down your throat so that the lining of your stomach can be seen.

Stomach biopsy... in which a small sample of tissue is taken from the stomach or small intestine which is examined in a medical laboratory for evidence of gastroparesis.

Non-intrusive methods:

Electrogastrography... is a test in which electrodes are attached to your skin to measure the electrical activity in your stomach which can be interpreted for gastroparesis.

Ultrasound... is a test in which sound waves are used to show the inside of your body.

Unfortunately, once any of these tests confirm that you do indeed have gastroparesis there is no cure. However you can manage the condition and its symptoms.

Diet changes to control gastroparesis

One of the best ways to control gastroparesis is through your diet. There are several things you can do:

Frequency: eat smaller meals but eat more often. Instead of three regular meals a day, eat six small meals. This way you will have less food in your stomach and it'll be easier for the food to leave your digestive system.

Texture: choose liquids, such as soups and broths, and other soft foodstuffs that are easy to digest. For example, eat pureed rather than solid fruit and vegetables.

Fats: avoid foods that are high in fat which tends to slow down digestion.

Diet: follow the beating diabetes diet... ie eat natural, unprocessed foods, mainly plants, that are... low in sugar... low in fat... low in salt... high in fibre... digested slowly... but excluding: all dairy products and eggs. You also need to drink plenty of water, to aid the absorption of the fibre you eat which can tend to slow down the passage of food through your stomach.

These simple adjustments to your diet will get your blood glucose levels under control and should also prevent your gastroparesis from getting any worse.

Treatments for gastroparesis

Certain medications can make gastroparesis worse. These include drugs for high blood pressure, anti-depressants, and certain medications for diabetes. You need to discuss this matter with the staff in your diabetes clinic, to see if you can have them changed.

There are several drugs that can be used specifically to treat either the cause or the symptoms of gastroparesis. However most of them have unwanted side effects.

Certain drugs can help move food along your digestive system:

Metoclopramide ... increases muscle contractions in the upper digestive tract which helps food pass through your digestive system quicker. It may also prevent nausea and vomiting. You take this drug before you eat. Its side effects include diarrhoea.

Erythromycin... an antibiotic, also causes your stomach to push food along. Its side effects too include diarrhoea.

Domperidone... is another drug that increases the transit of food through the digestive system. It can also relieve the nausea and vomiting associated with gastroparesis. Its side effects include headache.

Other drugs can also help prevent nausea and vomiting:

Dimenhydrinate... is an antiemetic used in the treatment of the symptoms of motion-sickness, ie nausea and vomiting. It is available as an over-the-counter antihistamine in most jurisdictions. Its side effects include drowsiness and mucus in the lungs.

Ondansetron... is a drug that blocks the chemicals in your brain and stomach that cause nausea and vomiting. Its side effects include headache, fatigue, and constipation.

Prochlorperazine... is another medication that helps control nausea and vomiting. Its side effects include drowsiness, dizziness, blurry vision, skin reactions, and low blood pressure.

In extreme cases of gastroparesis, surgical intervention may be necessary:

Gastric electrical stimulation... uses a surgically implanted pacemaker-like device (a gastric pacer) with electrical connections to the surface of the stomach that sends brief, low-energy impulses to stimulate the contraction of the muscles that propel food through the stomach. This decreases the duration of satiety and may also help reduce nausea and vomiting.

Feeding tube placement... in extreme cases, a tube can be inserted through the abdominal wall directly into the small intestine. In this case the patient is fed special liquid meals through the tube.

Not a pleasant prospect.

Gastroparesis develops slowly over the years. It can be avoided if you get your blood glucose levels under control and the best way to do this is to follow the beating diabetes diet.

NATURAL RELIEF FROM DIABETIC AUTONOMIC NEUROPATHY COMPLICATIONS

Diabetic autonomic neuropathy (DAN) is a complication of diabetes that affects the entire autonomic nervous system [ANS] causing significant negative impact on both survival and quality of life. Because the ANS serves the major organ systems of the body (e.g., cardiovascular, gastrointestinal, genitourinary, sweat glands, or eyes), any disorder affecting it is experienced as a body-wide dysfunction in one or more organ systems.

The ANS which is responsible for the involuntary functions of the human body is made up of the parasympathetic nervous system which controls the dynamic state [homeokinesis] of the body at rest to regulate the body's "rest and digest" functions while the sympathetic nervous system controls the body's responses to a perceived threat as in the "fight or flight" or emergency response.

The vagus nerve controls the lungs, heart and digestive tract thereby influencing the primary functions of breathing, speech, keeping the larynx [voice box] open during breathing, sweating, monitoring and regulating the heartbeat, satiety, and emptying of the stomach. Thus, when diabetes damages to the vagus nerve it causes loss of innervations and physiologic functions to the anatomic parts of the body it serves.

The esophageal dysfunction in DAN is directly related to vagal neuropathy. The main effects involve swallowing difficulties and heartburn. The heartburn is due to a relaxation of the esophageal sphincter which allows stomach contents to backup into the esophagus causing a burning pain in the chest following eating, bending down and or while lying down at night.

Today's food technology developments have allowed for the development of blenders that we can use to do the 'chewing' of food for us. We can use these blenders to make 'smoothies' which require minimal effort to swallow. This puts less demand on esophageal muscles during swallowing and thereby mitigates the effects of DAN.

Every cell in the human body is primarily designed to run on metabolizing glucose, the end product of carbohydrate digestion to meets its energy requirements. Thus, intimate knowledge of carbohydrate metabolism can help us manage the process from its intake to elimination. Carbohydrates have the advantage of a high fiber content which slows down the rate of glucose absorption to avoid blood glucose overwhelm. Modifying carbohydrate intake by making smoothies out of vegetables and fruits significantly helps us up our raw vegetable intake which helps manage blood sugar.

Autonomic neuropathy in diabetics slows the emptying of stomach contents, due to a partial paralysis [gastroparesis] which in turn leads to other problems such as fermentation of food in the stomach. Diabetic gastroparesis is diagnosed in about 25% of diabetic patients. Typical symptoms are premature feeling of satiety, nausea, vomiting, regurgitation, abdominal fullness, epigastric pain and anorexia. When the food is processed is such ways that allows it to be easily digested and released, the usual presentation of pain associated with it are ameliorated.

The gastric signs of DAN arise from a dilation of the stomach plus the retention of its content. This dilation of the stomach interferes with satiety feedbacks to the brain especially in cases where there is severe acidosis or coma. Green smoothies generally have alkaline pH; this will neutralize the acidosis to prevent the premature satiety feedback to the brain.

Constipation when it is observed is often associated with the compaction and compression of food into hard pellets which can create problems of absorption in the intestine and subsequently form hardened feces. When we employ a blender to make smoothies, the vegetables and fruits are thoroughly chewed allowing for easy digestion and prevent constipation.

DAN causes diffuse and widespread damages of peripheral nerves and small vessels. This is critically important because it is at the level of these small blood vessels called capillaries that transfer of nutrients from the blood to the cells occur. Stabilizing blood sugar will minimize the damage to peripheral nerves and blood vessels.

Individuals with DAN tend to have increased heart rate of 120-130 beats per minute compared to about 60 to 100 times per minute for normal persons at rest. Increased heart rate is associated with dizziness, lightheadedness, angina (chest pain) and shortness of breath. Another symptom experienced by diabetics with DAN is a postural hypotension in which the subject experiences a head rush or dizzy spell upon standing up or stretching. The combined cardiovascular responses mean the diabetic would have a slow reaction time designed to avoid precipitating a critical episode when responding to emergency events around him or her.

Another feature commonly associated with DAN is one of exercise intolerance in which the patient is unable to do physical exercise at the level or for the duration that would be expected of someone in his or her general physical condition. Healthcare providers very often advice diabetics to alter their lifestyle which is a euphemism for exercise. One hears phrases like 'don't be a couch potato' thrown around often but the physiological presentations of postural hypotension and exercise intolerance explains why persons with DAN show no interest whatsoever in taking up the exercise advice.

TYPE 2 DIABETES - DIGESTION AND DIABETES

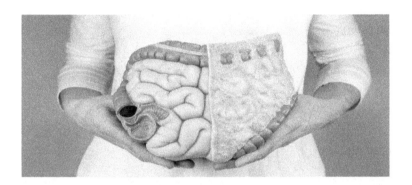

When Type 2 diabetes strikes, almost every system and area of your body is affected at some level... with some systems being disrupted more than others. While some of these areas might only be mildly impacted, it doesn't diminish the fact they are not operating at optimal efficiency. But other areas are much more dramatically impacted. As a result, the person diagnosed with Type 2 diabetes has to not only deal with their diabetes, but the many other life-altering side effects that have been created because of it.

One of these areas which is greatly impacted is digestion. This is due to autonomic neuropathy and involves the nerves whose functions are more or less automatic... those that control:

the stomach,

sweat glands,

digestive tract,

intestinal system,

bladder,

penis, and

circulatory system.

Gastroparesis, a neuropathy-related digestive problem, can include symptoms of nausea, diarrhea, or constipation... to name a few.

Medications can give relief for most symptoms of gastroparesis, as can such simple changes in eating habits as eating smaller meals more often and also adjusting the amount of fiber in your diet.

Also known as paralysis of the stomach, gastroparesis occurs when the vagus nerve, or the central nerve responsible for crushing food into particles which can be easily digested, becomes damaged. Once the vagus nerve is damaged, food is not broken down properly and, therefore, it cannot mix with the appropriate enzymes for processing. This means the stomach doesn't empty normally and naturally, food is then not absorbed. These processes are also impacted negatively by a high-fat meal.

When the normal digestive process is interrupted, the individual will then experience a long list of uncomfortable symptoms. They can have:

diarrhea,

nausea,

abdominal pain,

constipation,

vomiting,

bloating,

a feeling of fullness,

heartburn,

weight loss. or

a combination of some or all of these symptoms.

Even if stomach acids and digestive enzymes are released as intended, they will still contribute to the side effects due to the fact the food has not been adequately processed for digestion.

Unfortunately, this is not the end of the problems as blood sugar levels will also be affected dramatically. When food is unable to be digested, it makes it incredibly difficult to control your blood sugar levels. Since the body is not receiving the necessary vitamins and nutrients from the food, the body is not able to receive what it needs in order to have balanced blood sugar.

But the trouble does not stop there. When blood sugar levels are not balanced, it unfortunately also means the gastroparesis worsens. This ensures the vicious cycle continues. This is why it is important to keep gastroparesis away to start with.

If a person with Type 2 diabetes begins to experience problems as an aftermath of eating, they should consult with their doctor immediately.

Type 2 diabetes is no longer a condition you must just live with. It need not slowly and inevitably get worse. Now is the time to take control of the disease... and take back your health and your life.

PAIN, REFERRED PAIN AND DIABETES

Nobody likes pain and it can occur in any part of your body, at any time. However, pain doesn't always originate in the spot where you actually feel it. You often get referred pain. This is when a spot feels painful but the pain is being referred from another point in your body.

For example, if you have neck pain, it may be caused by general muscle tightness in your upper back. If you have a massage, your upper back needs to be worked on as well as your neck, in order to ease the pain. If your neck is the only spot worked on, the pain may ease a little but it will return as the area causing the pain was not attended to.

If you are having a heart attack, you may get referred pain in your neck, arms and shoulder. If you have pain in your throat, that can cause referred pain in your ear. If you eat icy cold food, you may experience what's known as "brain freeze" and this causes a bad headache because the coldness chills your vagus nerve.

If you get referred pain from your spine, it's generally because a nerve or a nerve root has become compressed. Causes include:

muscle spasms,

disc problems,

tumors,

fractures of the spine, or

osteoarthritis.

Referred pain is more common in older people but it can strike at any age. Trauma can cause referred pain for anybody.

Symptoms of referred pain from the thoracic and cervical spine include:

weakness in the muscles,

poor coordination, especially in your fingers and hands,

tingling and/or numbness in your hands and fingers, and

pulsing pain in your chest, arm, shoulders or neck.

Naturally, the actual location of symptoms will depend where the problem originates from. If you put your hands on your head, you may be able to temporarily ease the pain as this increases the amount of space between your cervical vertebrae.

When nerves become compressed, they cannot send out the same messages as they would normally and that's why you may get numbness and tingling. Other nerves carry "motor" function messages and, if affected, your muscles can become weakened and you may find it hard to coordinate your movements properly.

Diabetes makes pain worse because high and unstable blood sugar affects your nerves. This means you can suffer from referred pain more often due to nerve damage.

If you have pain:

consult a physical therapist to help determine the exact nature of the problem and the best means to correct it.

also consider your posture. Leaning over a desk all day, can cause additional pressure on certain parts of your spine, leading to compression if continued for long periods of time.

Pain of any type is unpleasant. If it's referred pain, it can be harder to treat and this is why it's essential you seek help to correct any problems before they get worse.

Type 2 diabetes is not a condition you must just live with. By making easy changes to your daily routine, its possible to protect your heart, kidneys, eyes and limbs from the damage often caused by diabetes, and eliminate some of the complications you may already experience. Maintaining a healthy blood sugar level means avoiding nerve damage.

TYPE 2 DIABETES: CAUSE AND CURE

Type 2 diabetes information can be extremely misleading. Not long ago, it was believed that type 2 diabetes could not be reversed. By 2013, a number of nutrition scientists had spent years researching a cure for type 2 diabetes, and all of them came to the same conclusion: type diabetes can be cured.

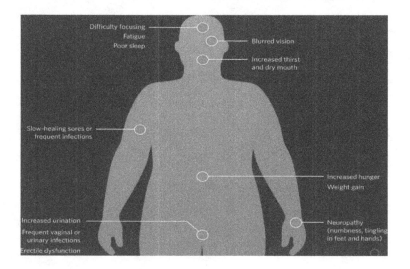

Many experts estimate that by the year 2040 1 out of 8 people, potential staggering 1.16 billion people, will be diabetic.

According to Statistics Canada, in 2013, almost 2.0 million Canadians had been diagnosed with this condition. The Public Health Agency of Canada cites a prevalence rate among adults of 8.7%, or one in 11 Canadians. In the US, the figure for 2012 was 29.1 million, or 9.3% of the population, plus an additional 86 million Americans who are per-diabetic.

One acquires the condition when insulin secreted by the pancreas is not able to transport all the excess sugar to the cells to be used as energy to fuel the muscles. This is known as insulin resistance, a condition increasing so dramatically that the World Health Organization (WHO) has put together an action plan to help bring diabetes under control.

With billions spent each year by diabetics and even more spent on prevention and treatment by developed nations worldwide, why is diabetes still on the increase?

It is not uncommon to hear even academics accept the notion that the condition should be managed. The astonishing thing is that there is no scientific evidence or proof that the condition cannot be reversed-yet most diabetics have accepted what is not their fate and resigned themselves to living with diabetes. But should they? Should they make a decision based old and outdated belief system?

We can draw a parallel between this condition and the planetary system. In the 60s and 70s, we were taught in schools that there were nine planets in our solar system, and we believed it for decades. Fast forward to 2010, by which time astrophysicists had estimated that there were 100 billion galaxies in the universe and that each galaxy could have 100 billion planets. Some astronomers say there are so many galaxies that they have stopped counting.

Had they made such statements back in the 60s, they would have been laughed at. Just as much as we now know that there are billions of galaxies in our solar system, we now know that type 2 diabetes is reversible and curable condition. For example, when I was diagnosed in 2009, at age 46, my blood glucose level was 21.9 millimoles per litre or 394.6 milligrams. (The normal level is 4.0 to 5.9 mmol/L, trending up to 7.8 mmol/L after meals.) There was so much sugar built up in my body that it had begun to exit as a sticky white substance on my tongue and at the corner of my eyelids each morning. My physician, Dr. Anthony Robinson, cautioned him, "Do you know the danger you have put yourself in? You are not far from going into cardiac arrest." Even with such compromised health, by working with both Western and Eastern doctors and through extensive research, I reversed my condition in less than three weeks simply by restoring his body's insulin sensitivity.

The condition caused by a lifestyle. In this way, it is like obesity. It is well known that if you consume too many calories, you gain weight. If the same eating habit continues, the weight gain may progress to what is called overweight and finally obese.

This condition follows a similar path. If a person ignores the early signs, eventually he or she will acquire the condition. If the person insists on ignoring the condition by continuing the same lifestyle choices, then his type 2 diabetes, which is curable, may progress to type 1 diabetes, the incurable type.

There are two types The type 1 and 2. Ninety percent of diabetics are type 2. Type 1 accounts for the remaining 10%. While type 2 is curable, type 1 is incurable.

Your body needs energy to function properly. Your brain needs energy to function. All this energy comes from the sugars that the body converts from carbohydrates we eat. As it was explained previously, you become type 2 diabetic when your body becomes insulin-resistant.

To reverse the condition, all you have to do is restore your body's sensitivity to insulin. This is accomplished using several approaches so that they all work together, according to Dr. Anthony Robinson and other Western and Eastern medical doctors. But if your blood cells are coated with fat, how can they absorb and use the sugar they need for energy? The solution is rather tricky.

When you engage in various physical activities, your body requires energy to fuel you. If it cannot get energy from your blood cells, it has no option but to use your body fat for energy. As your body begins to use fat for energy, it will use also use the fat that covers your red blood cells. This makes it possible for your red blood cells to absorb the sugars they need to give you energy.

SYMPTOMS OF DIABETES

A simple blood test will reveal if you have diabetes or not the test looks at the concentration of glucose in the blood stream and this is then measure against the glycemic index which will determine which carbohydrates have the highest levels of concentration of both sugars and starches that prove difficult for many diabetics to digest. Diabetes is normally broken down into two categories when someone is first diagnosed they are classed as either Type 1 or Type 2 diabetes. As a whole they are more generally adults. Some people may discover that they have Type 2 diabetes when they just feel off color and not well for no particular reason.

The signs that are most common that would signal further investigation are frequent urination, unquenchable thirst or drinking above what they normally would drink and this could be accompanied by an increased appetite. Mistakenly the symptoms that present could in some cases in the beginning look like the start of a cold or some other illness therefore symptoms of diabetes may be overlooked initially. Further symptoms such as fatigue, is a symptom of Type 1 diabetes with an unexplained weight loss even though you might have been eating more.

What is happening is that the glucose concentration in the blood (glycemia) is raised beyond the normal indicators and the glucose remains in the urine which then causes more pressure on the kidneys and results in further urination. Left unchecked diabetes can lead to kidney damage.

Many people with Type 1 diabetes may present with nausea, stomach pain and at times could result in a comatose state. A diabetic coma which can result when diabetes is undiagnosed can possibly result in death.

The simple solution is that you should make an appointment to see your Dr to investigate these vague symptoms. The other type of diabetes is Hypoglycaemia which is when the patient has below normal amount of glucose in the blood. These symptoms are at times varied but could include fainting, feeling off color even coma. Even so the more sensible thing that your Dr could request is a blood test to diagnose if you have either high or low blood sugars and to investigate any abnormal blood glucose.

Today Doctors know more about diabetes than ever before and depending which Type diabetes you have will determine the treatment and once you start the treatment prescribed you will be able to control the disease.

Remember, if you have a family of history of diabetes, or are overweight get a your blood sugar tested today in order to get the right treatment and if you experience any of the symptoms mentioned above do not delay make an appointment to see the Dr today.

THE BEST TYPE OF DIABETES DIET

For some, changing your diet can be one of the most difficult processes you will face while controlling our diabetes. The good new is there is not one specific type of diabetes diet. You have a variety of ways to practice healthy diabetic eating and still enjoy the food you eat.

Being committed to healthier eating and controlling your blood sugar begins in your mind. Just like the old saying goes, "If you think you can, you can. If you think you can't, you can't. There is much truth to that statement. You must make up your mind to take control. If you don't take control of your diabetes the consequences could be brutal and even life threatening.

For me, just thinking about the complications caused by poor diabetes control is enough to motivate me to choose healthy nutrition for diabetes. Blindness, heart disease, kidney failure, and amputations are all primary complications of diabetes. The sad part is that if a person just makes the conscious decision to eat a healthy diet and get regular exercise, the number of these complications could be drastically reduced. Avoiding these horrible complications takes daily management...not just an occasional thought of diabetes control. Eating to control your diabetes rewards you with a much healthier body, and thus allows you to live your life as you choose rather than as your diabetes and health allows.

Understanding Healthy Food Choices

Eating a health diet for diabetes doesn't require a specific type diabetes diet. Today there is not one set diabetic diet. You'll find more than one way to control your food intake to help you control your diabetes. Eating healthy for diabetes involves portion control, and balancing your intake of each of the three main food categories, carbohydrates, fats, and proteins. Of the three main food categories, carbohydrates, fats, and proteins, carbohydrates have the most impact on your blood sugar levels.

Good nutrition for diabetes begins with a basic understanding of how what you are eating affects your diabetes and your blood sugar ranges. Balancing food with your activity levels and your diabetes medications or insulin will help you get your blood sugars closer to a normal range blood sugar. Of the three main food categories, carbohydrates, fats, and proteins, carbohydrates have the most impact on your blood sugar levels.

In general eating no more than 45 to 60 carbohydrates per meal is recommended. Try to stay away from processed foods and refined carbohydrates. These foods don't contain the same vital phytonutrients as fresh fruits and vegetables. Processed foods and refined carbohydrates can also cause a spike in blood sugars, making them more difficult to control. Portion control is vital to healthy eating for diabetes. Watching serving size and not overeating will help to control blood sugar as well as help to manage weight.

HOW TO REVERSE TYPE 2 DIABETES NATURALLY

Diabetes is one of the most popular diseases affecting people around the world. It is a condition which causes your blood sugar levels to become higher than usual. Diabetes can be categorized into Type 1 and Type Diabetes with the latter being the most common.

What is Type 2 Diabetes?

This is a chronic condition which makes your body fail to use the insulin it produces appropriately. Insulin is responsible for regulating the movement of sugar into your cells. With type 2 diabetes, instead of the body converting sugar into energy, it stores it in the bloodstream.

The difference between type 2 Diabetes and type 1 diabetes is that the latter is caused by inadequate insulin in the body due to the immune system in some people destroying the cells that generate insulin. Unlike type 2 Diabetes, a person's lifestyle doesn't contribute to the development of type 1 diabetes which makes it hard to prevent..

Why Type 2 Diabetes Occurs

This type of diabetes occurs due to the body cells becoming insulin resistance where they ignore to take sugar from the blood. When there is too much sugar in your bloodstream for a prolonged period, muscle and fat cells will ignore the directions of insulin to take sugar from the blood hence more sugar accumulation in your bloodstream. Under normal condition, your pancreas produces adequate insulin to drive sugar into your cells. However, during the development stage of type 2 diabetes, your cells ignore to take sugar hence the sugar continues to move freely in your bloodstream. This forces the pancreas to produce more insulin to try to maintain the normal sugar levels but fails to keep up with the pace in the long run. The excess sugar in your body is sometimes converted and stored as cholesterol which is why most victims of this diabetes type are overweight. Inactive lifestyle, smoking, poor diets are the main factors associated with the development of this diabetes condition. The disease can also be hereditary. Although the disease can affect a person of any age, people at their early to mid-forties are at higher risk of getting this condition.

What It's Like On A Day To Day Basis For People Living With Diabetes Type 2

People living with type 2 diabetes are most likely to experience increased hunger, fatigue, hand and feet numbness, excessive thirst, and urge to urinate frequently. Blurred vision, weight loss, and slow healing of infections other symptoms that people with diabetes suffer from. These symptoms develop gradually such that some people will not note the change in life and will not even know they are suffering from this condition. This condition is progressive and may result in devastating effects if it is not controlled on time. Over time, high sugar levels in the bloodstream can cause damage to small blood vessels and nerves of the eye, kidneys or worse the heart. Large arteries are at high risk of hardening which can result in heart failure and stroke. Frequent urination may result in excessive loss of water in the body making one to be dehydrated. The kidneys are also forced to work harder which can cause them to fail. In the worst condition, type 2 diabetes can lead to organ failures resulting in amputation. Staying under medication is a struggle people who have Type 2 Diabetes have to endure every day for the rest of their life.

Treatment For Diabetes Type 2

If you, a family member or a friend is diagnosed with type 2 diabetes, you will be glad to know there are some treatment means that can control or even reverse the condition.

Diet And Exercise Treatment Approach

The first approach to treating type 2 diabetes is following a healthy diet and exercising regularly to keep your body fit. Exercising makes your body use high amounts of energy hence the need to process more sugar. If more sugar is processed, there will be no excess sugar roaming in your blood. When it comes to diet, one should avoid a high intake of proteins and fats and instead make complex Carbohydrates a large part of your meals. Such carbohydrates include whole grains, potatoes, and pasta. You should also take meals regularly in small amounts to ensure gradual sugar release into the bloodstream. If one maintains a healthy lifestyle, you can easily fight the disease without using drugs.

Medication Approach And Managing Type 2 Diabetes

Even though the above treatment approach is simple and easy to follow, one may not be sure it will work hence the need for medication. Drugs are mostly administered to make the body more responsive to insulin. Below are some of the drugs that people have to take to survive when they have diabetes type 2.

Metformin andquot; This drug works by reducing the amount of sugar released by the liver and decreasing rate of sugar absorption in the digestive tract. This automatically lowers blood sugar levels hence sensitizes cells to insulin. However, this drug may cause bloating, nausea, abdominal pain, and diarrhea.

Sulfonylureas and quot; This drug works by boosting insulin production. However, they may fail to work after some time, cause weight gain, and abnormally decrease sugar levels.

Biguanides andquot; These drugs function by decreasing the amount of glucose produced in the body. The side effect of this drug includes weight loss.

Megalitinides andquot; These drugs are taken before meals with the aim of boosting the production of insulin. Their impact is short-lived even though they give immediate effects. They can cause low blood sugar levels and make one to gain weight.

Thiazolidinediones - These drugs work by enabling body cells to accept insulin. They can, however, cause a heart attack. SGLT2 inhibitors - They work by preventing re-absorption of sugar into the blood by the kidneys by instead get rid of it in urine. They can, however, cause low blood pressure, vaginal yeast infections, diabetic ketoacidosis, and Urinary tract infections. Regardless of their side effects, these drugs are good for patients at risk of heart attack or stroke.

DPP-4 Inhibitors andquot; They block the functionality of dipeptidyle peptidase IV enzyme hence lowering sugar levels in the bloodstream. Their side effects include joint pain and pancreatitis.

GLP-1 receptor agonists and quot; These are injections that work by slowing metabolic rate hence lowering blood sugar. They can cause weight loss, pancreatitis, and nausea.

The decision to use drugs may be influenced by various factors which include blood sugar level and other health issues you may have, among others. Finding the ideal treatment for diabetes type 2 may require seeking medical advice. You may be required to combine various drugs to control your disease.

Does one have to endure taking the above drugs for a lifetime? Is it possible to reverse diabetes type 2? Well, there are some programs out there made to help people suffering from Type 2 Diabetes that treat the condition naturally. One such program is The Big Diabetes Lie.

The Big Diabetes Lie. This is a 456 pages book written by Max Sidorov and The International Council for Truth in Medicine (ICTM). It contains strategies on how to reverse Type 2 Diabetes naturally. If you have diabetes, the book promises to deliver you from the slavery of medications through a procedural health guide called The 7 Steps to Healthy and the Big Diabetes Lie.

How It Works

The program enlightens the users about everything to do with Type 2 diabetes right from how it develops and how to fight it. With this program, one learns about the adjustments they can make in their lifestyle to keep them safe from not only type 2 diabetes but also from other diseases. The program poses the question to the reader are your current diet choices keeping you diabetic? Some of the lessons one will learn from this book include healthy foods and the ones to avoid, choice of vitamins, differentiating healthy fats from the unhealthy ones, and how to reduce food craving among others. The book also teaches one how to maintain the appropriate PH level to make your body unfriendly to diseases like cancer. Overall, the guide emphasizes on healthy eating and lifestyle routines as the key to controlling and even reversing type 2 diabetes and preventing an attack from other diseases.

The Big Diabetes Lie claims the pharmaceutical industry is out to exploit the people living with Type 2 diabetes. Based on the authors' argument, the industry is after profit by selling drugs that they know can't completely treat Type 2 Diabetes but insist one cannot survive without their usage. The big pharmaceutical companies are afraid that other successful approaches will affect their bottom line and put them out of business. According to the authors, drugs treat symptoms instead of getting rid of the disease's root cause and even causes more life-threatening side effects compared to those of the disease itself. This is evident in the above drugs since none of them lacks a side effect.

Why It Is Successful

Unlike the drugs which only address the symptoms of Type 2 diabetes, this program tackles the root cause of the problem to make the patient free forever. It teaches you how to reverse type 2 diabetes naturally. Drugs are just meant to profit the pharmaceutical industry. The guide also uses natural strategies and will not cause any ill effects to the user. The program has worked for thousands of people around the world and maybe your solution too.

Type 2 diabetes is majorly a lifestyle disease. Even though there are other contributing factors, poor lifestyle is the main culprit. Educating people about this disease is the first step to fighting it. How do we inform the victims and prevent others from being diagnosed? Understanding everything about the condition is the key. The above guide outlines practically everything about this disease. There should be public awareness of what people should eat, how they should exercise, control their weight, and change their lifestyle. Most people have a hectic life and have little or no time to exercise. To make the matter worse, they are consuming junk foods in high amounts hence making them easy prey for type 2 diabetes. With proper education on how to observe a healthy lifestyle, Type 2 Diabetes can become history. This could be the diabetes breakthrough that saves your life.

DIABETES - THE CHRONIC KILLER

Diabetes mellitus or DM is a disease affecting multi-organ systems due to the abnormal insulin production, improper insulin usage or even both. It is a very serious health problem throughout the world effecting thousands of people.A survey conducted in United States showed that almost 6.2% of the population suffers from this disease. It is a matter of great issue that almost one -third of the population is unaware of the disease.

Incidence

Diabetes is actually the fifth leading cause of deaths in the country of United States. And the real incidence is expected to have a steady increase in the coming years. Diabetes has a very important role in leading to heart disease, adult blindness, stroke, non traumatic amputation of lower limb etc. it is found that diabetic people do have a risk of almost two fold to develop coronary artery disease and that too with more than 65% suffering from high blood pressure.

Diabetes - a short review

Diabetes mellitus are of mainly three types, they include type 1 diabetes mellitus, type ii diabetes mellitus, gestational diabetes and also secondary diabetes. Gestational diabetes as its name refers to deals with the diabetic episode during pregnancy or during the gestational period. It will subside once after delivery. Secondary diabetes is another form of diabetes where diabetes will occur secondary to other diseases, for instance chronic hypertension.

Type I diabetes mellitus or juvenile diabetes

It is known as juvenile diabetes since it is more common among the juveniles or young people below 30 years of age. It is insulin dependent diabetes with a peak onset during the age group of 11 to 13. Type I diabetes is caused due to the progressive destruction of pancreatic beta cells that occurs by the auto immune mechanism. Clinical symptoms include increased frequency in urination or polyuria, excessive thirst or polydipsia, increased hunger or polyphagia, weight loss, fatigue etc are seen. Ketoacidosis is a very serious complication seen in children due to diabetes and is often life threatening and may lead to metabolic acidosis.

Type II diabetes mellitus

Over 90% of diabetes mellitus is type ii diabetes.here the pancreas continues to produce insulin,but this amount of insulin is either poorly used up by tissues or is either inadequate for bodily needs. There are mainly three abnormalities or factors leading to type ii diabetes mellitus. One of them is insulin resistance, where insulin receptors are either minimal in number or will remain unresponsive. Another factor is the poor ability of pancreas to produce insulin. The final factor comes with inappropriate glucose production by the liver.

Risks related to diabetes

When we analyze the analyze risk group for developing diabetes mellitus, a condition that requires primary importance is impaired glucose tolerance or IGT. It is a disease condition caused by the mild alteration of beta cell function. Here the blood glucose level is usually high but not to a level to be called as a case of diabetes. But most people with impaired tolerance for glucose have a high risk for developing type ii diabetes within the next 10 years.

Another important risk related to diabetes is insulin resistance syndrome, also known by the name syndrome x,it is in fact a cluster of abnormalities which will act in a synergistic manner so a stop increase the risk of cardiovascular disease. It is usually charactracterised by increase insulin levels, high amount of triglycerides, hypotension.

Once identified, then complete cure of the disease is not so easy though proper measures can help you to control diabetes in a very effective way. Though there are many environmental as well as genetic factors involved in causing diabetes, exercises. Balanced diet, adequate rest and sleep and a stress less life could help you to keep away from diabetes or to stop diabetes.

There are a lot of management measures for diabetes control. It chiefly includes nutritional therapy, exercise therapy, oral anti-glycemic agents, insulin treatment etc. therefore a collaborative management is usually preferred for treating diabetes mellitus. Nutritional therapy is one of the main management for diabetes mellitus.

Diabetic diet

Diabetic diet management is one of the main components of the collaborative management. Some of the general guidelines for diabetic diet include the following.

Fiber rich diet: Always include the fiber rich food in the diet as it could increase the bulk of your stomach and can add on to your satisfaction.

Restrict sodium intake up to even 2400mg/dl.

Include whole grains, fresh fruits and vegetables in the diet.

There is an alternative mode of planning the diabetic diet which is considered as one of the convenient method. This often referred as plate method. The most important advantage of this method is that here the patient itself could visualize the amount of starch, vegetables, and whatever food filled in the nine inch plate.

For lunch and the dinner, half of the plate is to be filled with non starchy vegetables, one fourth with starch and another one fourth with any non vegetarian items up to 2-4 oz. A single glass of milk with low fat and a small piece of fresh fruits could complete the meals.

When we look on to the breakfast, the plate has to be filled with starch around half and another one forth with optional proteins.

This plate method is found to be very useful as it could owe about 1200-1400 cal/day, which adds on to an appropriate balanced diet plan.

Nutritional therapy can do much to control diabetes. But there is a small variation in the diet plans of patient s with type I diabetes and type ii diabetes. When we consider total calories, type I diabetic people needs increased calorie intake because it commonly occur in young people and therefore for the proper maintenance and restoration of tissues, diet with good calorific value is important. While in the case of type ii people, this is often restricted for obese or overweight people.

Effect of diet is very much crucial in type I diabetes as not only food control but also insulin therapy is also a must in type I diabetes. Uniform timing for meals is considered very strict in the case of type I diabetes mellitus because of the multi doses of insulin's but this is just desirable for type II diabetes mellitus. If needed, intermittent snack can be taken for diabetic patients with type I form, though it is not much recommended for type II diabetes. Usually the frequent snack is not recommended for type diabetic people.

It should very seriously note that diet teaching should not only focus on the patients but also to his family and caregivers. It is most suitable to give adequate teaching to the person who is cooking and serving. But still, the ultimate responsibility to maintain their blood glucose fall on to the patients. Try to avoid alcohol also since it could again worsen your body and health by causing hyper glyceridemia. Besides all these, regular exercises, strict drug regime, periodic screening etc should be done to control diabetes and its effects. Diabetes if monitored and maintained in a very appropriate way, it could be effectively controlled.

DIABETIC AMYOTROPHY

Diabetic amyotrophy is a diabetic neuropathy that usually occurs to type 2 diabetic patients. There is a lot of pain and numbness and muscles weakness, most especially in the thigh, hip and buttocks. This condition mostly happens to middle aged women and older men who have type 2 diabetes. This condition has also been referred as the Bruns-Garland Syndrome, proximal diabetic neuropathy and lumbosacral radiculoplexus neuropathy.

Diabetic amyotrophy is extremely painful. It usually happens in the night and could attack one side of the body at a time. Although pain is usually concentrated in the middle part of the body and upper limbs, pain could also travel and extend to the toes, legs, feet, hand and arms. Some of the early signs of diabetic amyotrophy are numbness to pain and extreme temperature, tingling, burning and prickling, cramps, sensitivity to touch and loss of coordination and balance.

One could also observe feet deformities, blister and sores on the numb areas. These should be treated immediately as infection from the sores could extent to the bones. Infected bones will need to be amputated to prevent from spreading all throughout the body. This is a very severe effect of diabetes which is very common to happen.

So what is diabetes? Diabetes is a metabolic disease wherein the patient has high blood sugar level due to low insulin or inability to respond to the insulin produced by the body. Classic diabetes symptoms are constant thirst, hunger and frequent urination. There are several types of diabetes:

• Type 1 - Also referred to as juvenile diabetes or insulin-dependent diabetes. This happens when the body fails to produce insulin, thus the patient's need for regular insulin shots. It usually occurs suddenly on thin children.

• Type 2 - This is the so-called adult-onset diabetes or the non-insulin dependent. This is the resistance of the body to use the insulin that is naturally produced. This is developed gradually among obese adults.

• Gestational Diabetes - This happens to otherwise healthy women who have developed high glucose level in the blood during pregnancy. This could develop into Type 2 diabetes if left untreated.

Aside from these three types, diabetes can also be due to genetics, monogenic, due to cystic fibrosis or induced by excessive use and dosage of steroids. Both Type 1 and Type 2 diabetes are incurable. Symptoms can be hold in check with insulin shots and proper Type 1 and Type 2 diabetes diet.

Aside from the genetic factors, type 2 diabetes is caused by excessive and abusive lifestyle. Among the prime contributors are smoking, alcoholic intake and a diet contradictory to the ideal type 2 diabetes diet. To avoid the risk of acquiring type 2 diabetes, one must stay away from foods that are fatty and with high sugar contents.

The diabetic amyotrophy can last as long as five months if left untreated. To get relief from the pain, the patient should immediately seek the help of a doctor. The patient will have to undergo a thorough physical examination to determine the overall condition of the patient. He will then be advised of the best diet, exercises, insulin shots if needed and other medications. These are all aimed to lower the glucose level in the blood, which caused the diabetic amyotrophy.

SYMPTOMS OF DIABETES

Diabetes mellitus is a persistent illness in which your blood glucose levels are too high. Cells in your body break down the sugar in order to provide vigor for movement, increase, and renovation of life. The hormone insulin is in charge for regulating sugar levels in the blood.

Excessively high levels of glucose can harm the large and small blood vessels, leading to blindness, kidney illness, amputations of limbs, stroke, and heart ailments. These are the three most common kinds of diabetes:

1 - Type 1 diabetes is typically, though not always, diagnosed in children and young adults. People with type 1 diabetes produce no insulin and must take it each and every day.

2 - Type 2 diabetes is habitually diagnosed in adults over 45 years old. In this type of diabetes, either you are not producing enough insulin, or your body is dead set against insulin and cannot use it suitably. As many as 50 percent of people with type 2 diabetes are unaware that they have this condition. That is why it is particularly important to take notice of the signals and symptoms and its menace factors.

3 - Gestational diabetes: expecting women who have never had diabetes previously but who have high blood glucose levels for the period of pregnancy are said to suffer from gestational diabetes. This form of diabetes affects about 4% of all pregnant women. It may herald advance of type 2 (or seldom type 1) diabetes.

KEEP YOUR EYES OPEN TO IDENTIFY THESE DIABETES SYMPTOMS

A few of the signs of either type diabetes are: being extremely thirsty, losing the sensation in your feet or having tingling in your members. In type 1, symptoms often increase over a short interval of time. Take into account that the most frequent symptoms in younger children are weight loss, polydipsia (excessive thirst), and polyuria (urinating a lot).

In type 2, diabetes symptoms build up more gradually, and some people never have any symptoms of the ailment. Symptoms of type 2 diabetes comprise being overweight and suffering from acanthosis nigricans, a velvety itchiness on a child's neck. If you are regularly having any of these symptoms, you should tell your medical doctor. Most people who are diagnosed with diabetes have type 2 diabetes.

IT MIGHT BE NOT TOO LATE

If you are fated to develop type 2 diabetes you might live many years in a situation of prediabetes, termed "America's largest healthcare epidemic", a condition that occurs when your blood sugar levels are very high but not enough for you to be diagnosed with type 2 diabetes. As of 2009 there are nearly 60 million persons who suffer from prediabetes in the USA alone.

Other types of diabetes mellitus are usually categorized independently from the above mentioned. Examples might include:

* Innate diabetes - due to hereditary defects of insulin emission,

* Cystic fibrosis-related diabetes,

* Some sorts of monogenic and steroid diabetes, caused by high doses of corticoids.

THE TYPES OF DIABETES - TREATMENTS AND FOOD

Diabetes is the forth disease which affects greater number of people in world. Each year, about 380 thousand people die by diabetes. In India after every 10 seconds one patient dies because of diabetes. This number may increase up to 38 million, in year 2025. These numbers equal the number of people dying of HIV/AIDS and malaria. The patients do not get proper treatment because of lack of awareness. The patients have to maintain the sugar level in their blood.

Beta cells and islets of Langerhans produce insulin in human body, which is affected because of diabetes. This disease is found in women more than men. An interesting fact about diabetes is that most of the patients affected by this disease are not aware. They realized about the fact when they go for the check up of some other disease.

At present there are 24 million diabetics. Now the people get affect by diabetes in age of 15-20 years. As compared to earlier times the age limit for this disease is decreasing rapidly. The main causes of diabetes are overweight, improper life-style, fast-food and lack of physical exercises.

Insulin for diabetes:

Some patients think that insulin is not needed, which is not right. In diabetes there are most of the conditions when it become necessary to give insulin. Insulin is helpful in balancing blood sugar level. Some of the patients think if they once take insulin they have to take it regularly, also they think that their kidney will be affected by insulin. Some of the patients change their doctors because of this illusion.

Diabetes type:

Diabetes type 1:

The human body cannot create insulin in proper manner because of diabetes type 1. This type of diabetes is mostly found in kids and youth. It is one type of auto immune disorder, which is caused because of inability of pancreas for creating insulin. For the people suffering from diabetes type 1 it is necessary to take insulin for a normal life. Diabetes type 1 is more harmful than other types of it. Actually less than 10% of diabetics fall under this category. The patient feels increased hunger and thirst and becomes under weighted. The diabetes type 2 cannot be obliterate completely but can be controlled up to 58% by following a proper life-style and a proper diet.

Diabetes type 2:

Mainly adult and old age people get affected by diabetes type 2 but now a days teen-age rs also get affected by it because of improper life-style. Body of the patient of diabetes type 2 creates insulin but cannot absorb it and hence the level of sucrose increases in the blood. The patients of diabetes type 2 become over weight. The 90% of diabetics fall under this category and out of them 80% are overweight. If the patient does not get proper treatment on time, it may result into other major problems like heart, kidney, eye and nerve related diseases.

Home Remedies for diabetes:

avoid starchy food,

use less oil,

eat vegetables like spinach,

avoid white bread, potatoes and sweets,

avoid coffee and alcohol.

ALL DIABETES ARE NOT THE SAME

In my previous chapter, I helped you better understand the problems and solutions of diabetes type 1. Unfortunately, many Americans suffer from another type of diabetes that is far more prevalent and this chapter will help you better comprehend the differences. Here's a general description on the two types:

Diabetes falls into the category of metabolic diseases characterized by high blood sugar levels. Under normal conditions, blood glucose levels are controlled by insulin, a hormone produced by the pancreas, the organ responsible for sugar control. All types of diabetics have difficulty either producing too much or not enough. Here is the difference between type 1 and type 2 diabetes in a nutshell.

o Type 1 diabetes is sometimes called juvenile diabetes and occurs when the pancreas stops producing insulin. Nobody knows exactly why this happens, but some experts believe a virus or an autoimmune response, in which the body attacks its own pancreatic cells, is responsible. People with this type of diabetes must take insulin for life.

o Type 2 was once known as adult-onset and those affected are noninsulin-dependent. In the case of type 2 diabetes, the pancreas secretes plenty of insulin, but the body's cells don't respond to it.

Age, Gender, and Obesity Linked to Type 2 Diabetes

Did you know that men, aged 35 to 54 are almost twice as likely to have diabetes as women? Recent studies indicate that although diabetes occurs in people of all ages and races, some groups have a higher risk for developing the disease. What researchers don't know is why certain people develop type 2 diabetes and others do not.

What medical reports do tell us are the factors that increase a person's risk of getting type 2 diabetes. Let's take a look at the relationship of type 2 diabetes and three very important characteristics that put you in danger of developing the disease.

o Weight - The more fatty tissue you have, the more resistant your cells become to insulin.

o Inactivity - Physical activity helps you control your weight, uses up glucose as energy and makes your cells more sensitive to insulin.

o Age - The risk of type 2 diabetes increases as you get older, especially after age 45. It may be because as people age they tend to become less active, lose muscle tone and gain unwanted weight.

Its no wonder these common risk factors have sparked concern among members of the medical profession.

More Staggering Statistics

You might agree that it seems more and more people you know are becoming a statistic; one more victim of diabetes 2. I'd like to share a few facts about this fast growing disease that might be of interest to you.

o Type 2 diabetes is the most common form and is responsible for 90% - 95% of the 21 million people afflicted with the disease.

o People over 40 are at higher risk of the condition, as are people with a large waist or family history of the disease.

o Type 2 diabetes is the form linked to poor exercise and diet. Many of the two million people with type 2 are overweight or obese - and an estimated 500,000 more people have type 2 but do not know it.

o The number of obese people will increase in the coming decades, putting people at higher risk of heart disease, stroke and certain types of cancer.

o Type 2 diabetes can be undetected for a decade or longer and many already have complications by the time it is diagnosed. These complications include heart disease, stroke, kidney failure, blindness and amputation.

The News Is Not All Bad

If you have been diagnosed with type 2 diabetes it might seem frightening at first. But don't let it get you down. Although type 2 diabetes is serious, it is also manageable. If you are willing to follow a healthy life style you can reduce your risk of developing the disease as well as learn to control it. Consider this:

o Losing weight can reduce the risk of type 2 diabetes in high-risk people by 58 percent.

o Exercising can cut the risk by 64 percent.

There are also natural remedies for type 2 diabetes that are being explored in addition to standard treatment. Make sure that you inform your doctor about any herbs, supplements, or natural treatments you are taking to safeguard against adverse reactions with other medications.

Diabetes Improves With Natural Minerals

o Chromium is a mineral that helps increase the efficiency of insulin, and picolinateis an amino acid that allows the body to use chromium much more readily.

Research shows that chromium picolinate helps lower blood sugar levels in most type 2 diabetics after taking a daily supplement containing the mineral. What's even better is chromium picolinate has shown to reduce obesity which means it may enable some people with type 2 diabetes to lose enough weight to stop taking drugs entirely.

o Magnesium is a mineral that can be found naturally in green leafy vegetables, nuts, seeds, and whole grains. It is needed to help regulate blood sugar levels as well as other bodily functions. Some studies suggest that magnesium supplementation may improve insulin sensitivity and lower fasting glucose levels.

o Zinc is important to type 2 diabetics because it helps in the production and storage of insulin. It can be found naturally in oysters, ginger root, lamb, pecans, split peas, egg yolk, rye, beef, liver, lima beans, almonds, walnuts, sardines, and chicken.

o Vanadium can be found in soil and many foods and has been found to improve insulin and reduce blood sugar. It actually imitates the action of insulin in the body.

COPING WITH TYPE 2 DIABETES DISEASE

Numerous individuals are examined and diagnosed with type diabetes each and everyday. Diabetes has unfortunately become one of the most prevalent diseases to affect individuals in the world today. When an individual is diagnosed with type 2 diabetes they might get a feeling of being bewildered and overpowered because of the diagnosis. It is crucial then for individuals who are diagnosed with type

2 diabetes to understand and comprehend that with some rudimentary alternations in their life style and with careful monitoring coping and living with the disease is totally achievable.

Learning About Type 2 Diabetes

The initial consideration an individual that has type 2 diabetes needs to do is to start to become educated and familiar with their disease and it effects on their body, different complications and ways to get it under control to as much extent as possible. The doctor should assist the patient by starting with some rudimentary instruction and be ready to recommend additional resources of information for the individual. The diabetic should talk to a dietitian that is registered and with a diabetes educator that is certified to further educate themselves about the disease.

Changes In Diet

The person who has been newly diagnosed with diabetes will have to get counseling through a registered dietitian. The dietitian can guide the type 2 diabetic to educate themselves in regards to the foods that they eat and what necessary modifications can be made for the best result to their body functions. There are also many different types of cook books as well as websites that offer recipes for diabetics that will enable a person to consume healthy tasty meals. The diabetic will need to address their dietary changes seriously.

Watching Blood Sugars

The type 2 diabetic will have to get a glucometer so they will be capable of monitoring their blood sugar on a day to day basis within there home. There are numerous different types of glucometers that you can get on the open market today that are highly accurate provided that the person uses them in a correct way. The majority of insurance companies will furnish a monitor with the initial diagnosis of type 2 diabetes. By monitoring closely their own blood sugar levels an individual can in a relatively easy manner see what kinds of foods as well as their activities are giving the biggest effect and make any needed changes accordingly.

Type 2 Diabetic and Exercises

A very helpful thing for any individual, particularly a type 2 diabetic to do is to establish some kind of exercise program. One of the direct results of exercise is the decrease of the levels of blood sugars. You do not have to have a highly complex type of exercise routine to accomplish what you need to. The person with diabetes can just start out with walking, biking or a swimming regimen. Going for a walk around the neighborhood several times each week will be very beneficial to the overall health of the diabetic in addition to lowering their blood sugar levels.

Taking Medications

The type 2 diabetic should follow all of the advice of their doctor and take their medications as they are prescribed to them. There are numerous types of excellent medications that function very well to control diabetes when working in conjunction with exercise and dietary changes. Type 2 diabetics have to take any and all medication that are necessary in their individual circumstances to stabilize the blood sugars and maintain a high quality of life.

HEALTHY TIPS FOR DIABETES

Diabetes is a very serious health concern for many people who are diagnosed with this disease. Statistics indicate that diabetes is surging in the US due to many factors. By 2050 diabetes can affect as much as 30% of the population. At present, over 20 million Americans have diabetes and millions remain unaware that they too have the disease. Sadly, there is also a growing rise in children being diagnosed with diabetes, something that was almost unheard of a few decades ago. Having diabetes also appears to increase your risk of developing cancer as well. Medical costs to care for diabetes cost the US over 175 billion per year. That astronomical amount is indicative of the state of poor health we are facing as a nation. Estimates say that over 60% of adults are considered obese, a key factor in developing diabetes. This doesn't take into account the tragic side effects associated with diabetes such as kidney failure, heart disease, and amputations from infections.

Diabetes Defined: Diabetes is caused when the body fails to secrete insulin properly from the pancreas. Insulin helps sugar to reach the body's cells in order to create energy. When insulin levels aren't working properly it effects sugar levels and diabetes can develop. There are two types of diabetes; Type 1 and Type 2. Type 1 diabetes usually occurs in childhood. It is more serious because it involves the immune system destroying pancreas cells that secrete insulin. This is about 10% of all diabetes. Type 2 is also known as "adult onset diabetes" because it predominantly affects adults. The pancreas cells improperly utilize insulin. This results in a cycle of producing more insulin to compensate. Eventually the body loses the ability to produce it, literally from "burn out". There are numerous medications that are used to help control diabetes but as of yet there is no cure. However, there are various natural healthy ways you can help yourself feel better if you are diabetic. Healthy lifestyle choices can also potentially prevent you from developing it in the first place. Of course you should always be under the care of a trained medical professional if you are diabetic and follow your doctor's instructions regarding prescriptions, diet and lifestyle.

Exercise: Exercise helps to improve the way your body utilizes insulin. By exercising you help your body burn fat and build muscle. Lower fat levels also help decrease blood pressure to normal ranges and reduce your risk of heart disease. You will also get the added benefits of more energy and strength. If your blood sugar levels are very high, always consult with your doctor before beginning any exercise programs.

Glycemic Index of Foods: The glycemic index of foods is a chart that shows how much insulin in involved in digestion. It indicates how a carbohydrate type food raises blood glucose levels. Foods with a high glycemic index are unhealthy choices for diabetics. You should plan your meals around foods that have a low to medium glycemic index. Balance any high GI foods with low GI foods to balance out the meal. Low GI foods that are good choices include non starchy vegetables and whole grain breads. Protein foods such as meats and fats don't have a GI Index because they do not contain carbohydrates. There is much reason to believe that diabetes is a modern day disease brought on in large part by diet and lifestyle in its type 2 form. When cultures switched from a plant based high fiber diet to the westernized high fat sugar filled type, diabetes became a commonplace illness. Our eating habits are very poor and we are literally inducing disease through poor nutrition. Research indicates we could reduce type 2 diabetes by 50% if we incorporate exercise and reduced sugar in our diets.

Resveratrol: The skin of red grapes contains a very powerful substance known as "resveratrol". These polyphenols help control glucose levels in the body. What does this do? It prevents spiking in blood sugar levels which is what diabetics experience as part of the disease. Nutritionists recommend one glass of wine with dinner or supplementing with a high quality resveratrol capsules. Research indicates that type 2 diabetes is directly related to how much fat is in the bloodstream. The higher the fat the more likely diabetes can develop. It appears that resveratrol counteracts this fat and allows insulin to function properly.

Other Helpful Foods: Tumeric: This popular Indian spice is similar to curry in flavor. Tumeric has been widely studied and it appears to be beneficial to health in numerous ways. It may be helpful to diabetes as well as having liver cleansing properties. The main ingredient in turmeric, known as "curcumin" is what holds the key to the powerful benefits of turmeric. You can use this spice on your favorite meat and rice dishes to add a healthy zesty flavor. Omega 3 fatty acids: Fish that is high in omega-3 fatty acids may also be helpful. Best fish for omega-3 includes salmon, tuna and mackerel.

Dark chocolate may help reduce insulin resistance according to an Italian study conducted in 2006. However it must be dark chocolate, not the highly processed chocolates that we commonly eat. Eating foods such as blueberries and strawberries that contain antioxidant phytochemicals can also help reduce the risk of diabetes. Cherries contain one of the highest sources of anthocyanins. A 2004 animal study concluded that anthocyanin helped increase insulin production. Other fruits that contain anthocyanins include strawberries and red grapes. Other foods you may consider incorporating into your diet include beans which help stabilize insulin and blood glucose levels in the body. Of course eating a diet high in whole fresh vegetables and fruits, small amounts of lean protein and whole grains is an ideal choice for diabetics and for anyone wishing to prevent the development of this disease. Remember whenever beginning any dietary or lifestyle changes, always consult with a medical professional, particularly if you are taking prescription drugs or suffer from any disease or ailment.

WHY THE DIABETICS FOOD GUIDE
PYRAMID MAY BE DANGEROUS

The food guide pyramid was designed to help both Type I Diabetics and Type II Diabetics. In our country, the majority of diabetics are not showing signs of improvement. It isn't uncommon for a diabetic to follow their food guide pyramid, or their suggested program to the letter and still not see a change in their blood sugar levels.

You can type 'diabetic food guide pyramid' into Google or any internet search engine and get results. These generic, non-specific guides may work for you or may not. Some are misleading and some are very useful. Always remember that type two diabetic needs to be very careful when choosing which guide to follow.

The type two diabetic should learn that a guide that has the bottom section of the diabetic pyramid made up of grains, making it seem like grains are the most important food for diabetics, is very misleading. Some guides recommend; 6

servings or beans, grains and starchy vegetables like peas and corn.

The reality is that grains and starchy vegetables like peas and corn are heavy in carbohydrates. Carbohydrates are turned in to sugar once in the body. This can only damage the diabetic body, and therefore misleading as a food guide, and should never be followed blindly, without reason.

Also know that there are some people who will argue that whole grain foods are good for Type II Diabetics. Whole grain foods, while they are better for the human body then processed grains, are still high in carbohydrates. Following the advice of eating a daily diet of 6 servings of grains and starches would be dangerous to the health of most Type II diabetics, possibly leaving them with nearly no chance of recovery.

It would appear that the diabetes food pyramid is not effective in helping people with Type II diabetes. It is fairly common that those who do follow these types of food guides, without the proper supervision of a healthcare professional or physician, not only do not improve their condition, but in many cases worsen their condition as a result. There is a need for an effective food guide specifically designed to help diabetics improve their condition. Any diabetic knows how important diet is in controlling their Type II Diabetes. They need both useful and accurate information and right now, are having trouble getting it.

There are doctors that choose to educate their patients on the food types that can best help their condition. Type II diabetes is fast becoming an epidemic, while health care workers continue to recommend the same diet that they have seen fail over the years. As a whole, most people with Type II diabetes are getting worse, even while following the diabetes food guide pyramid or other programs like it.

As a diabetic, you should make it your goal to learn a system of diet that is easy to follow and recreate week after week, one that is designed to cater to your individual needs. Find a doctor that works with individual clients to find healthy foods that they enjoy and that they can easily make. There are a lot of healthy food recipes available.

FOUR STEPS TO CONTROL DIABETES

Diabetes is a serious disease, affecting all parts of the body.

STEP 1: Learn about Diabetes:

Diabetes means that blood sugar levels are too high. Here are the type (type) diabetes:

Type 1 diabetes: The body does not produce insulin. Insulin helps the body use sugar from food to produce energy. Type 1 diabetes who need insulin injections every day.

Diabetes type 2: decreased body produce and use insulin. Diabetes patients need to take pills or insulin. Diabetes type 2 Diabetes is a common one.

Diabetic pregnancy:

Occurs as the patient is pregnant increases the risk of another type of diabetes, especially type 2 diabetes. Increased risk of obesity and diabetes problems for children.

Diabetes is a very serious disease!

Take good care of yourself and Diabetes will help patients better and avoid complications such as:

* Cardiac arrest or stroke (cerebral vascular accident)

* Eye problems leading to disturbances of vision or blindness

* Damage to nerves cause stinging sensation, numbness cold, loss of sensation, wounds in hands and feet can lead to amputation.

* Complications of chronic kidney causing kidney failure.

* Gum disease and tooth loss causes....

When blood sugar levels near normal patient

* There are more energetic

* Less tired, thirsty and urinate less

* The healing of wounds and less prone to skin infections, urinary tract infection than

* Less problems with skin, eyes, feet.

STEP 2: Understand the overview Diabetes

Ask your doctor about controlling HbA1c, blood glucose, blood pressure and cholesterol. This will help reduce the risk of cardiac arrest, stroke and other complications of diabetes.

ABC of diabetes is an abbreviation of the following:

A's: (HbA1c): a test of red blood sugar:

HbA1c test will measure the average blood glucose of patients in the last 3 months. Goal for most patients is <7%.

Higher average blood sugar will cause complications to the heart, blood vessels, eyes, kidneys and feet

Letter B: a blood pressure (Blood pressure)

The patient's blood pressure diabetes is below 130/80 mmHg best.

High blood pressure makes the heart work exertion. It can cause complications: cardiac arrest, stroke and kidney disease.

Letter C: is Cholesterol

LDL-cholesterol targets of diabetes patients is <100 mg / dl and

HDL - cholesterol is> 40 mg / dl.

LDL-cholesterol is "bad" cholesterol, can fill and clog the blood vessels. This can cause cardiac arrest and stroke. Meanwhile, HDL-cholesterol is "good" cholesterol helps remove bad cholesterol from blood vessels

STEP 3: Diabetes Management

Patients can avoid complications by better care of themselves. Be good cooperation with your physician to achieve ABC.

Use this self-care program:

Dietary program for patients with diabetes:

Eat healthy foods such as fruits, vegetables, fish, lean meat, skinless chicken, dried peas or beans, whole grains (brown rice) milk for patients with diabetes and cheese.

Use the diet of fish, lean meats and poultry around 100 grams.

Eat foods low in fat and salt

Eat fiber-rich foods such as whole grains, bread, rice or noodles

Exercise regularly weekdays:

Daily physical activity should be set 30-60 minutes. Brisk walking is the exercise most effective and easily

Maintain ideal body weight, avoid obesity by choosing healthy foods and physical activity more.

Ask others for help if you see mental collapse.

Learning to cope with stress: Stress can increase blood sugar, so be reasonable to relax when feeling tense.

Quit Smoking

Take medicine regularly, even when feeling healthy. Tell your doctor if any side effects.

Check feet daily to see if there are cracks, skin blisters, red spots and swelling or not? Tell your doctor immediately if any unusual.

Measuring blood sugar:

The patient can measure blood glucose one or more times a day.

Measuring blood pressure checked

Report any changes to your doctor vision

STEP 4: Often going to the doctor to avoid medical complications

Each time the examination will be:

* Check blood pressure

* Check legs

* Test weight

* Check self-care programs such as step 3

HbA1c test every 2 years or more times if HbA1c> 7%

Each year should have at least 1 test:

* High blood cholesterol

* Blood Triglyceride

* Check your teeth, tell your dentist know diabetes

* Eye exams to detect complications in the eye

* Considering the urine and blood to test kidney function

IS TYPE II DIABETES REVERSIBLE?

Diets with unbalanced amounts of meat and dairy products are contributing to higher cholesterol levels and bigger waistlines. Unhealthful diets are the leading cause of heart problems and diabetes. Diabetes type II is weight onset. Is type II diabetes reversible? Three solutions to this question are offered below.

1. Is Type II Diabetes Reversible? Yes, with Bariatric Surgery

Bariatric surgery, also known as gastric bypass surgery. Surgery technique makes the stomach a smaller pouch and restricts food intake. Is type II diabetes reversible? Yes, this surgery improves glucose metabolism to normal levels just after one month of surgery.

2. Is Type II Diabetes Reversible? Yes, with Vitamin D (experimental)

One of the consequences of obesity is Vitamin D deficiency. According to Endocrine Today, "Obesity is associated with low vitamin D levels and low vitamin D levels have been associated with both insulin resistance and beta cell dysfunction." Is type II diabetes reversible? According to a recent study of type II diabetes in Endocrine Today, it "showed that vitamin D supplementation improved endothelial function." Endothelial is the endothelium made up of a layer of cells that line blood and lymph vessels, heart cavity and other serum organs. Endocine Today reports that "lowering insulin resistance vitamin D supplementation should have the potential of not only preventing type II diabetes but also of preventing cardiac events."

"It is possible that utilizing vitamin D supplements in the obese vitamin D insufficient or deficient subject would prevent the development of type diabetes," according to Endocrine Today. Is type II diabetes reversible? The answer to this question could be easily funded by a government agency or a vitamin D company. This could be one of the answers to an obesity pandemic as simple as it may sound.

3. Is Type II Diabetes Reversible? Yes, try Dr. Neal Barnard

Dr. Neal Barnard has a diabetes-reversing diet called, "Slim, Trim + Vegan." He is an author, clinical researcher, and health advocate. He has been investigator in many studies of diet and health, and especially in diabetes and diet. Dr. Barnard graduated from George Washington University School of Medicine in Washington, D.C. with a M.D. degree.

Three methods have been discussed of what others can do for you for type II diabetes reversal. You can also prescribe your own diet and exercise plan. The following tips explain how.

One of the best ways to lose weight is by diet and exercise and the right kind of both. According to clinical studies, one of the best items to include in your diet is soluble fibers, also known as PolyGlycopleX (PCX). PCX lowers your blood sugar level after a meal so you do not have a hungry feeling. In addition, PCX can help you lose weight. According to the Journal of the American Dietetic Association, a study "demonstrated that children who ate more soluble fiber had fewer diabetes risk factors, including obesity."

According to Mayo Clinic, the Mediterranean diet is a healthy choice. This heart-healthy diet includes fish, whole grains, vegetables, nuts, fruits, and health fats such as olive oil. You can even throw in some wine.

Whenever there is a change in diet, continue a consistent physical activity routine. The Diabetes Prevention Program study "demonstrated that 30 minutes of moderate exercise a day combined with a reduction in body weight of just 5 to 10 percent, produced a 58 percent decrease in diabetes risk."

Best Foods for Diabetes

If you have diabetes, it can be hard to figure out how to eat to feel your best and keep your blood sugar under control. But there are lots of diabetic diet-friendly foods you can enjoy. And rather than keeping the focus on what foods to avoid with diabetes, it's refreshing to focus on the foods you can and should be eating more of. These top foods to eat with diabetes are nutrient-packed powerhouses that can help you control your blood sugar and stay healthy.

Breakfast (360 calories, 40 g carbohydrates)

1 serving Strawberry-Orange Breakfast Cakes

1 clementine

A.M. Snack (154 calories, 20 g carbohydrates)

2 carrots

¼ cup hummus

Lunch (327 calories, 29 g carbohydrates)

1 serving Tomato Salad with Lemon-Basil Vinaigrette

Avocado Toast (1 slice whole-wheat toast + ½ avocado-mashed + 1 tsp. Sriracha)

P.M. Snack (141 calories- 17 g carbohydrates)

10: unsalted almonds

1 cup raspberries

Dinner (373 calories, 38 g carbohydrates)

1 serving Chipotle Chicken Satay with Grilled Vegetables

1/2 cup brown rice

Daily total: 1,355 calories, 145 g carbohydrates

Breakfast (331 calories, 29 g carbohydrates)

1¼ cups nonfat plain Greek yogurt

¾ cup raspberries

2 Tbsp. walnuts

1 tsp. honey

A.M. Snack (143 calories, 15 g carbohydrates)

2 celery stalks

1 Tbsp. unsalted peanut butter

1 clementine

Lunch (289 calories, 37 g carbohydrates)

1 serving Pulled Chicken & Pickled Veggie Wraps

1 cup strawberries

P.M. Snack (185 calories, 17 g carbohydrates)

5 whole-wheat crackers

1 oz. reduced-fat Cheddar cheese

Dinner (408 calories, 45 g carbohydrates)

1 serving Better-Than-Takeout Burgers with Sweet Potato Fries

Daily total: 1,357 calories, 143 g carbohydrates

Breakfast (296 calories, 41 g carbohydrates)

1 serving Coconut-Cashew Breakfast Bites

1 clementine

A.M. Snack (156 calories, 18 g carbohydrates)

1 cup sugar snap peas

¼ cup hummus

Lunch (375 calories, 33 g carbohydrates)

1 serving Grilled Salmon Salad with Raspberry Vinaigrette

2 carrots

P.M. Snack (145 calories, 19 g carbohydrates)

10 unsalted almonds

1 peach

Dinner (351 calories, 45 g carbohydrates)

1 serving Sheet Pan Orange-Apricot Drumsticks

1 cup mixed greens

1 Tbsp. balsamic vinegar

Daily total: 1,323 calories, 156 g carbohydrates

Breakfast (336 calories, 31 g carbohydrates)

1¼ cups nonfat plain Greek yogurt

1 cup sliced strawberries

2 Tbsp. walnuts

1 tsp. honey

A.M. Snack (146 calories, 15 g carbohydrates)

1 Tbsp. unsalted peanut butter

2 carrots

Lunch (329 calories, 40 g carbohydrates)

1 serving Chicken Potpie with Cauliflower Topping

2 clementines

P.M. Snack (139 calories, 15 g carbohydrates)

¼ cup part-skim mozzarella cheese

3 sliced tomatoes

Basil leaves

Dinner (365 calories, 49 g carbohydrates)

1 serving Broccolini, Chicken Sausage & Orzo Skillet

½ cup raspberries

Daily total: 1,314 calories, 150 g carbohydrates

Breakfast (271 calories, 42 g carbohydrates)

1 slice whole-wheat toast

1 Tbsp. unsalted peanut butter

1 sliced banana

A.M. Snack (135 calories, 16 g carbohydrates)

1 cup raw green beans

¼ cup hummus

Lunch (378 calories, 55 g carbohydrates)

1 serving BLT Pizza

P.M. Snack (176 calories, 17 g carbohydrates)

1 hard-boiled egg

5 whole-wheat crackers

Dinner (392 calories, 44 g carbohydrates)

1 serving Raspberry-Pineapple Fish Tacos

1/4 cup low-sodium canned black beans

Daily total: 1,351 calories, 174 g carbohydrates

1. Cinnamon

This fragrant spice has been shown to lower cholesterol and keep blood sugar more stable. Just 1/4 teaspoon of cinnamon per day improved fasting blood sugar and cholesterol levels in one study published in the journal Diabetes Care, and other studies have shown similar effects. Get your cinnamon fix by sprinkling it into smoothies, yogurt, oatmeal or even your coffee. Another plus for cinnamon? It adds flavor to your food without adding sugar or salt.

Nuts

Walnuts in particular have been shown to help fight heart disease and can improve blood sugar levels, all thanks to walnuts' high levels of polyunsaturated fats. These healthy fats have been shown to help prevent and slow the progression of conditions like diabetes and heart disease.

Almonds, pistachios and pecans also contain these beneficial fats. Nuts are low in carbohydrates and high in protein and fat, which makes them good for stabilizing blood sugar. Just be sure to watch your serving size. A 1/4-cup portion of shelled walnuts clocks in at 164 calories.

Oatmeal

Whole grains, such as oats, are better for your blood sugar (the fiber helps minimize spiking) and may actually help improve insulin sensitivity. Oats contain fiber in the form of beta-glucans, which are the soluble fibers that cause oats to bulk up in liquid. Soluble fiber regulates blood sugar by slowing down the breakdown and absorption of carbohydrates from other foods you eat. Studies have also shown oats can help improve blood pressure, cholesterol and fasting insulin levels.

Dairy

In addition to providing calcium and vitamin D for healthy bones, dairy foods are an excellent source of protein to keep hunger at bay. Milk, cheese and yogurt have all been shown to help stabilize blood sugar levels, and eating plenty of these dairy products may reduce the risk of developing diabetes. New research suggests you don't necessarily have to stick to fat-free dairy. A large analysis from researchers at Harvard and Tufts found that eating more full-fat (or whole) dairy was associated with a lower risk of developing diabetes. It might be that the higher fat content keeps you feeling full, so you'll be less likely to reach for a sugary, high-carb snack later on. But, keep in mind that full-fat dairy is higher in calories than fat-free. Whether you choose fat-free or full-fat dairy, it's most important to watch for added sugars in flavored yogurts and milks, which can add significant calories in the form of simple carbs.

Beans

Beans are loaded with fiber and protein to keep you feeling full. Beans are also a source of carbohydrates, with about 20 grams of carbs per half-cup serving. One Canadian study showed that people who added a cup or more of beans to their diets every day had better control of their blood sugar and lowered their blood pressure. Beans are inexpensive and incredibly versatile. Mix things up by adding different varieties, such as black, pinto, garbanzo or cannellini beans, to veggie-packed salads and soups.

Broccoli

Broccoli-and other cruciferous foods, such as kale, cauliflower and Brussels sprouts-all contain a compound called sulforaphane. This anti-inflammatory compound helps control blood sugar and protects blood vessels from damage associated with diabetes. Broccoli is not only low in calories and carbs-1 cup of cooked chopped florets has just 55 calories and 11 grams of carbohydates-but it also packs a lot of nutrients, including vitamin C and iron. You can feel free to fill half your plate with this good-for-you green veggie.

Quinoa

This protein-rich whole grain is a great substitute for white pasta or white rice. It contains 3 grams of fiber and 4 grams of protein per 1/2-cup serving of cooked quinoa. The boost of fiber and protein means quinoa gets digested slowly, which keeps you full and stops your blood sugar from spiking. Quinoa is also considered a complete protein, because it contains all nine essential amino acids, needed to build muscle, which is rare for plant-based protein sources. Plus, it's rich in minerals, such as iron and magnesium.

Spinach

Spinach is one of the best sources of magnesium, which helps your body use insulin to absorb the sugars in your blood and manage blood sugar more efficiently. This leafy green is also high in vitamin K and folate, among other key nutrients. Plus, a 2-cup serving of raw spinach delivers only 2 grams of carbohydrates and 14 calories. Munch on raw baby spinach in salads, add it to your morning smoothie or sauté it with garlic and olive oil for a healthy side dish.

Olive Oil

This Mediterranean-diet staple packs a punch when it comes to managing diabetes, mostly due to its high monounsaturated fatty acid, or MUFA, content. Several studies have shown that a diet high in MUFAs helps keep blood sugar in check by lowering insulin resistance, helping cells better respond to your body's insulin. There's no need to fear the fat from olive oil. While fat has more calories than carbohydrates, gram for gram, it helps keep you full, minimizes blood sugar spikes and allows your body to absorb key nutrients, such as vitamins A and E.

Salmon

Not only is salmon high in protein, it's also rich in omega-3 fatty acids, which can help keep your heart healthy by lowering blood pressure and improving cholesterol levels. Other types of fatty fish that contain omega-3 fatty acids, such as tuna, mackerel and sardines, can also provide these protective effects, which are especially important for people with diabetes, who are also at a greater risk for cardiovascular disease.

The Best 30-Day Diabetes Diet Plan

DAY 1

Chicken & Vegetable Penne with Parsley-Walnut Pesto

Homemade pesto may seem daunting, but in this quick pasta recipe you can make a simple sauce in minutes while the pasta water comes to a boil. You can substitute frozen green beans and cauliflower for fresh; in Step 4, cook the frozen vegetables according to package directions before tossing with the pasta and pesto.

Ingredients

¾ cup chopped walnuts1 cup lightly packed parsley leaves2 cloves garlic, crushed and peeled½ teaspoon plus ⅛ teaspoon salt⅛ teaspoon ground pepper2 tablespoons olive oil⅓ cup grated Parmesan cheese1½ cups shredded or sliced cooked skinless chicken breast (8 oz.)6 ounces whole-wheat penne or fusilli pasta (1¾ cups)8 ounces green beans, trimmed and halved crosswise (2 cups)2 cups cauliflower florets (8 oz.)

Preparation

Bring a large pot of water to a boil. Place walnuts in a small bowl and microwave on High until fragrant and lightly toasted, 2 to 2½ minutes. (Alternatively, toast the walnuts in a small dry skillet over medium-low heat, stirring constantly, until fragrant, 2 to 3 minutes.) Transfer to a plate and let cool. Set ¼ cup aside for topping. Combine the remaining ½ cup walnuts, parsley, garlic, salt, and pepper in a food processor. Process until the nuts are ground. With the motor running, gradually add oil through the feed tube. Add Parmesan and pulse until mixed in. Scrape the pesto into a large bowl. Add chicken. Meanwhile, cook pasta in the boiling water for 4 minutes. Add green beans and cauliflower; cover and cook until the pasta is al dente (almost tender) and the vegetables are tender, 5 to 7 minutes more. Before draining, scoop out ¾ cup of the cooking water and stir it into the pesto-chicken mixture to warm it slightly. Drain the pasta and vegetables and add to the pesto-chicken mixture. Toss to coat well. Divide among 4 pasta bowls and top each serving with 1 Tbsp. of the reserved walnuts.

DAY 2

Spinach, Apple & Chicken Salad with Poppy Seed Dressing & Cheese Crisps

Ingredients (4 servings)

3 9-by-14-inch phyllo pastry sheets, thawed4 teaspoons extra-virgin olive oil plus 2 tablespoons, divided1 large egg white, beaten⅓ cup freshly grated Parmigiano-Reggiano cheese1 tablespoon fresh thyme leaves3 tablespoons buttermilk2 tablespoons honey1 tablespoon cider vinegar1 teaspoon poppy seeds½ teaspoon Dijon mustard½ teaspoon kosher salt5 cups baby spinach1½ cups shredded cooked chicken breast1 medium Gala apple, sliced

Preparation

Preheat oven to 350°F. Line a baking sheet with parchment paper. Place 1 sheet of phyllo on the prepared baking sheet. Brush with 2 teaspoons oil. Top with a second sheet of phyllo, pressing gently to adhere. Brush with 2 teaspoons oil. Place the third sheet on top and brush with egg white. Sprinkle with cheese and thyme. Using a pizza cutter or sharp knife, cut the phyllo stack into approximately 2-inch squares. Bake until golden brown, about 8 minutes. Let cool for about 3 minutes. Meanwhile, whisk the remaining 2 tablespoons oil, buttermilk, honey, vinegar, poppy seeds, mustard and salt in a medium bowl. Add spinach, chicken and apple to the bowl and toss to coat. Serve with the phyllo crisps.

To make ahead: Refrigerate dressing (Step 3) for up to 2 days.

Equipment: Parchment paper

DAY 3

Hazelnut-Parsley Roast Tilapia

Sweet and crunchy hazelnuts team up with bright lemon and fresh parsley to add oomph to the tilapia for an easy seafood recipe. Serve this atop a salad or alongside brown rice or orzo.

Ingredients4 servings

2 tablespoons olive oil, divided4 (5 ounce) tilapia fillets (fresh or frozen, thawed)⅓ cup finely chopped hazelnuts¼ cup finely chopped fresh parsley1 small shallot, minced2 teaspoons lemon zest⅛ teaspoon salt plus ¼ teaspoon, divided¼ teaspoon ground pepper, divided1½ tablespoons lemon juice

Preparation

Preheat oven to 450°F. Line a large rimmed baking sheet with foil; brush with 1 Tbsp. oil. Bring fish to room temperature by letting it stand on the counter for 15 minutes. Meanwhile, stir together hazelnuts, parsley, shallot, lemon zest, 1 tsp. oil, ⅛ tsp. salt, and ⅛ tsp. pepper in a small bowl. Pat both sides of the fish dry with a paper towel. Place the fish on the prepared baking sheet. Brush both sides of the fish with lemon juice and the remaining 2 tsp. oil. Season both sides evenly with the remaining ¼ tsp. salt and ⅛ tsp. pepper. Divide the hazelnut mixture evenly among the tops of the fillets and pat gently to adhere. Roast the fish until it is opaque, firm, and just beginning to flake, 7 to 10 minutes. Serve immediately.

DAY 4

Charred Vegetable & Bean Tostadas with

Pile vegetables and black beans onto crisp tostadas and top them off with lime crema for a vegetarian dinner the whole family will love. Charring the vegetables under the broiler infuses them with smoky flavor while cooking them quickly.

.Ingredients 6 servings

Lime Crema5 tablespoons sour cream⅛ teaspoon lime zest2 teaspoons lime juice⅛ teaspoon kosher saltTostadas6 corn tortillas2 tablespoons canola oil plus 2 teaspoons, divided4 cloves garlic, sliced, divided1½ teaspoons ground cumin1 teaspoon kosher salt, divided⅛ teaspoon chipotle chile powder2 (15 ounce) cans no-salt-added black beans, rinsed¼ cup water, plus more as needed2 medium red bell peppers, sliced1 large red onion, halved and sliced2 medium zucchini, halved and sliced ½ inch thick1 cup fresh or frozen corn kernels¼ teaspoon ground pepper1 cup thinly shredded cabbage¼ cup chopped fresh cilantro6 tablespoons crumbled cotija cheese

Preparation

To prepare crema: Combine sour cream, lime zest, lime juice and salt in a small bowl. Set aside. To prepare tostadas: Position a rack in upper third of oven; preheat to 400°F. Brush both sides of tortillas with 1 tablespoon oil and arrange on a baking sheet. (It's OK if they overlap a bit; they will shrink as they cook.) Bake, turning once halfway, until browned and crisp, about 10 minutes. Transfer to a wire rack and let cool. Meanwhile, heat 2 teaspoons oil in a large skillet over medium heat. Add 1 garlic clove and cook, stirring occasionally, until fragrant, about 30 seconds. Add cumin, ½ teaspoon salt and chile powder; cook, stirring, for 30 seconds more. Add beans and cook, stirring occasionally, until heated through, about 4 minutes. Transfer the beans to a food processor and add ¼ cup water. Pulse until smooth, adding more water, 1 tablespoon at a time, if needed. Preheat broiler to high. Toss bell peppers, onion, zucchini, corn, ground pepper, the remaining 3 garlic cloves, 1 tablespoon oil and ½ teaspoon salt in a large bowl. Spread on a large rimmed baking sheet. Broil, stirring occasionally, until lightly charred, 8 to 12 minutes. Top the tostadas with some of the beans, charred vegetables, cabbage, cilantro, cheese and the reserved crema.

DAY 5

Pistachio-Crusted Baked Trout

Finely chopped pistachios take center stage in this baked fish recipe. Toasted seeds are mixed with the pistachios to create a fragrant and crunchy crust which nicely compliments the tender fish.

Ingredients4 servings

4 (4-5 ounce) fresh or frozen trout fillets (see Tip)½ teaspoon coriander seeds½ teaspoon cumin seeds½ teaspoon caraway seeds4 teaspoons olive oil1 teaspoon finely shredded lemon peel1 clove garlic, minced½ teaspoon kosher salt¼ teaspoon ground cinnamon¼ teaspoon ground pepper¼ cup pistachio nuts, finely chopped4 lemon wedges

Preparation

Thaw fish, if frozen. Preheat oven to 350°F. Line a shallow baking pan with foil and coat with cooking spray; set aside. Heat a small saucepan over low heat; add coriander seeds, cumin seeds, and caraway seeds. Cook and stir for 4 minutes or until fragrant and golden. (Do not allow the seeds to burn or they will taste bitter.) Remove from heat. Using a small food processor or a mortar and pestle, grind the seeds. Stir in oil, lemon peel, garlic, salt, cinnamon, and pepper. Place pistachios in a small bowl; set aside. Rinse the fish; pat dry with paper towels. Spread one side of the fish fillets with the spice mixture. Bringing up two opposite ends, fold the fish into thirds. Dip the top and the sides of the fish bundles into the nuts to coat; place in the prepared baking pan. Sprinkle with any remaining nuts. Bake for 15 to 20 minutes or until the fish begins to flake when tested with a fork (145°F). Serve with lemon wedges.

Tip: Save some time by asking your butcher or fishmonger to fillet the fish and remove the skin.

DAY 6

Pork Medallions with Cranberry-Onion Relish

Pork tenderloin is a great choice for dinner when it's thinly sliced into quick-cooking medallions. A tart cranberry and onion relish adds delicious taste to each bite of this 30-minute entree.

Ingredients

4 servings

12 ounces pork tenderloin¼ cup all-purpose flourPinch of saltPinch of ground pepper2 tablespoons olive oil, divided1 small onion, thinly sliced¼ cup dried cranberries¼ cup reduced-sodium chicken broth1 tablespoon balsamic vinegar

Preparation

Trim fat from pork. Cut the pork crosswise into eight slices. Place each slice between two pieces of plastic wrap. Using the flat side of a meat mallet, lightly pound the pork to ¼-inch thickness. Discard plastic wrap. Combine flour, salt, and pepper in a shallow dish. Dip the pork slices into the flour mixture, turning to coat. Coat a heavy large skillet with cooking spray. Add 1 tablespoon oil to the skillet; heat over medium-high heat. Add four pork slices to the hot oil; cook for 3 to 4 minutes or until the pork is slightly pink in the center, turning once halfway through the cooking time. Transfer the pork to a serving platter; cover with foil to keep warm. Repeat with the remaining 1 tablespoon oil and the remaining four pork slices. Cook onion in the same skillet over medium heat for about 4 minutes or until crisp-tender. Combine cranberries, broth, and vinegar in a small bowl; carefully add to the skillet. Heat through. Serve the onion mixture over the pork slices.

DAY 7

Lemon Chicken & Rice

This easy Persian-inspired chicken and rice dish has a beautiful golden color and a wonderful fragrance. If you have saffron in the cupboard, do add that optional pinch; just a little will enhance the flavor and aroma of the dish.

Ingredients

8 servings

2 tablespoons olive oil, divided8 boneless, skinless chicken thighs (1¼-1½ lbs. total), trimmed2 large onions, thinly sliced½ teaspoon salt, divided3 cloves garlic, minced2 teaspoons ground turmeric1 teaspoon paprikaGenerous pinch of saffron (optional)3 cups shredded cabbage (about ½ small head)4 cups cooked brown rice, preferably basmati or jasmine¼ cup lemon juice2 tablespoons chopped fresh Italian parsley (optional)1 lemon, sliced (optional)

Preparation

Prep

50 m

Ready In

1 h 35 m

Preheat oven to 375°F. Coat two 8-inch-square baking dishes or foil pans with cooking spray (see Tip). Heat 1 Tbsp. oil in a large nonstick skillet over medium-high heat. Add 4 chicken thighs, and cook, turning once, until both sides are lightly browned, about 4 minutes. Transfer the chicken to a plate and set aside. Repeat with the remaining chicken thighs. Pour off all but about 1 Tbsp. fat from the pan. Add the remaining 1 Tbsp. oil and onions to the pan and sprinkle with ¼ tsp. salt. Cook, stirring, until soft and golden, 12 to 15 minutes. Stir in garlic, turmeric, paprika, and saffron, if using; cook, stirring, for 2 minutes. Transfer the onions to a plate and set aside. Return the pan to medium-high heat and add cabbage. Cook, stirring, until wilted, about 3 minutes. Stir in rice, lemon juice, the remaining ¼ tsp. salt, and half of the reserved onion. Continue cooking until the rice is well coated and heated through, 5 to 7 minutes. Divide the rice mixture between the prepared baking dishes; nestle 4 of the reserved chicken thighs in each dish. Top each with half of the remaining cooked onions. Cover both dishes with foil. Label one and freeze for up to 1 month. Bake the remaining casserole, covered, for 30 minutes. Uncover and continue baking until a thermometer inserted in the thickest part of the chicken registers 165°F and the onions are starting to brown around the edges, 5 to 10 minutes more. Garnish with parsley and lemon slices, if desired.

Tip: Instead of freezing half, you can bake the full recipe in a 9x13-inch baking pan. In Step 6, bake, covered, for an additional 10 minutes.

To make ahead: This double-batch recipe makes one meal for tonight and one to freeze for up to 1 month (see Step 5). To cook from frozen: Thaw overnight in the refrigerator, then bake as directed in Steps 6-7, adding an additional 10 minutes baking time once uncovered.

Equipment: Two 8-inch-square baking dishes or foil pans

DAY 8

Pumpkin Seed Salmon with Maple-Spice

Because this one-pan meal is ready in just 35 minutes, it's a good choice for a healthy recipe after you've had a long day at the office. Maple-spiced carrots cook alongside pepita-crusted salmon fillets and deliver amazing taste and nutrition in a dinner the whole family will devour.

Ingredients

4 servings

4 (4-5 ounce) fresh or frozen salmon fillets1 pound carrots, cut diagonally into ¼-inch slices¼ cup pure maple syrup, divided½ teaspoon salt, divided½ teaspoon pumpkin pie spice8 multi-grain saltine crackers, finely crushed3 tablespoons finely chopped salted, roasted pumpkin seeds (pepitas) plus 2 teaspoons, dividedCooking spray

Preparation

Thaw fish, if frozen. Preheat oven to 425°F. Line a 15x10-inch baking pan with foil; set aside. Combine carrots, 3 tablespoons maple syrup, ¼ teaspoon salt, and the pumpkin pie spice in a large bowl. Arrange the carrots on one-half of the prepared baking pan. Bake for 10 minutes. Meanwhile, rinse the fish; pat dry with paper towels. Combine crushed crackers, 3 tablespoons of the pumpkin seeds, and the remaining ¼ teaspoon salt in a shallow dish. Brush the top of the fish with the remaining 1 tablespoon maple syrup. Sprinkle with the cracker mixture, pressing to adhere. Place the fish in the baking pan next to the carrots. Lightly coat the top of the fish with cooking spray. Bake for 10 to 15 minutes more or until the fish flakes easily when tested with a fork and the carrots are tender. To serve, divide the carrots among dinner plates and sprinkle with the remaining 2 teaspoons pumpkin seeds. Top with the salmon.

Salmon Couscous Salad

This healthy and easy salad is designed to be made with precooked or leftover salmon. To quickly cook salmon, lightly brush with olive oil, then roast in a 450°F oven until the fish is opaque and firm, 8 to 12 minutes.

Ingredients

1 serving

¼ cup sliced cremini mushrooms¼ cup diced eggplant3 cups baby spinach2 tablespoons white-wine vinaigrette, divided (see Tip)¼ cup cooked Israeli couscous, preferably whole-wheat4 ounces cooked salmon¼ cup sliced dried apricots2 tablespoons crumbled goat cheese (½ ounce)

Preparation

Coat a small skillet with cooking spray and heat over medium-high heat. Add mushrooms and eggplant; cook, stirring, until lightly browned and juices have been released, 3 to 5 minutes. Remove from heat and set aside. Toss spinach with 1 Tbsp. plus 1 tsp. vinaigrette and place on a 9-inch plate. Toss couscous with the remaining 2 tsp. vinaigrette and place on top of the spinach. Place salmon on top. Top with the cooked vegetables, dried apricots, and goat cheese.

Tip: To make a quick white-wine vinaigrette, whisk 2 Tbsp. white-wine vinegar with ⅛ tsp. each salt and pepper. Slowly whisk in ¼ cup extra-virgin olive oil until blended. Extra dressing will keep, covered, in the refrigerator for up to 5 days. Bring to room temperature before using.

DAY 9

Vegan Cauliflower Fettuccine Alfredo with Kale

Ingredients

6 servings

½ cup fresh whole-wheat breadcrumbs, toasted1 tablespoon chopped fresh parsley½ teaspoon grated lemon zest4 cups cauliflower florets (1 small head)1 cup raw cashews8 ounces whole-wheat fettuccine4 cups lightly packed thinly sliced kale3 tablespoons lemon juice2 tablespoons white miso2 teaspoons garlic powder2 teaspoons onion powder¾ teaspoon salt1 cup water

Preparation

Put a large pot of water on to boil. Combine breadcrumbs, parsley and lemon zest in a small bowl. Set aside. Add cauliflower and cashews to the boiling water; cook until the cauliflower is very tender, about 15 minutes. Using a slotted spoon, transfer cauliflower and cashews to a blender. Add pasta to the boiling water and cook, stirring occasionally, for 10 minutes. Add kale and cook until the pasta is just tender, about 1 minute more. Drain; return the pasta and kale to the pot. Add lemon juice, miso, garlic powder, onion powder, salt and 1 cup water to the blender; process until smooth. Add the sauce to the pasta and stir until well coated. Serve topped with the breadcrumb mixture.

DAY 10

Curried Sweet Potato & Peanut Soup

In this flavorful soup recipe, sweet potatoes simmer in a quick coconut curry, resulting in a creamy, thick broth punctuated by notes of garlic and ginger. We love peanuts for their inexpensive price and versatile flavor. They're also a great source of protein—1 ounce has 7 grams.

Ingredients

6 servings

2 tablespoons canola oil1½ cups diced yellow onion1 tablespoon minced garlic1 tablespoon minced fresh ginger4 teaspoons red curry paste (see Tip)1 serrano chile, ribs and seeds removed, minced1 pound sweet potatoes, peeled and cubed (½-inch pieces)3 cups water1 cup "lite" coconut milk¾ cup unsalted dry-roasted peanuts1 (15 ounce) can white beans, rinsed¾ teaspoon salt¼ teaspoon ground pepper¼ cup chopped fresh cilantro2 tablespoons lime juice¼ cup unsalted roasted pumpkin seedsLime wedges

Preparation

Heat oil in a large pot over medium-high heat. Add onion and cook, stirring often, until softened and translucent, about 4 minutes. Stir in garlic, ginger, curry paste, and serrano; cook, stirring, for 1 minute. Stir in sweet potatoes and water; bring to a boil. Reduce heat to medium-low and simmer, partially covered, until the sweet potatoes are soft, 10 to 12 minutes. Transfer half of the soup to a blender, along with coconut milk and peanuts; puree. (Use caution when pureeing hot liquids.) Return to the pot with the remaining soup. Stir in beans, salt, and pepper; heat through. Remove from the heat. Stir in cilantro and lime juice. Serve with pumpkin seeds and lime wedges.

Tip: You can find red curry paste in the Asian section of many grocery stores, packaged in a small glass jar.

To make ahead: Refrigerate soup for up to 3 days. Reheat before serving.

DAY 11

Spinach & Strawberry Salad with Poppy Seed Dressing

Homemade poppy seed dressing pairs beautifully with tender spinach, crunchy almonds and juicy berries for a fantastically refreshing and easy spring salad. To make ahead, whisk dressing, combine salad ingredients and store separately. Toss the salad with the dressing just before serving. To make it a complete meal, top with grilled chicken or shrimp.

Ingredients

4 servings

2½ tablespoons mayonnaise1½ tablespoons cider vinegar1 tablespoon extra-virgin olive oil1 teaspoon poppy seeds1 teaspoon sugar¼ teaspoon salt¼ teaspoon ground pepper1 (5 ounce) package baby spinach1 cup sliced strawberries¼ cup toasted sliced almonds

Preparation

Whisk mayonnaise, vinegar, oil, poppy seeds, sugar, salt and pepper in a large bowl. Add spinach and strawberries and toss to coat. Sprinkle with almonds.

DAY 12

Slow-Cooked Pork Tacos with Chipotle Aioli

Follow this pork taco recipe as is to serve four and you'll have enough shredded pork leftover to make it again next week. It's so good, however, that we recommend doubling the rest of the ingredients and inviting over four more friends to enjoy everything right away!

Ingredients

4 servings

1 (2 to 2½ pound) boneless pork sirloin roast3 tablespoons reduced-sodium taco seasoning mix1 (14.5 ounce) can no-salt-added diced tomatoes, undrained1 cup shredded romaine lettuce1 cup chopped mango⅔ cup thin bite-size strips, peeled jicama½ cup light mayonnaise2 tablespoons lime juice2 cloves garlic, minced½ to 1 teaspoon finely chopped canned chipotle pepper in adobo sauce (see Tip)8 (6 inch) corn tortillas, warmed¼ cup coarsely chopped fresh cilantro

Preparation

Prep

40 m

Ready In

4 h 10 m

Trim fat from roast. Sprinkle with taco seasoning mix; rub in with your fingers. Place the roast in a 3½- or 4-quart slow cooker. Add undrained tomatoes; cover and cook on Low for 7 to 8 hours or on High for 3½ to 4 hours. Remove the roast, reserving cooking liquid. Shred the meat using two forks. Toss the meat with enough cooking liquid to moisten. Set half of the meat aside (about 2½ cups) and place the remainder in an airtight container for later use (see Tip). Combine lettuce, mango, and jicama in a medium bowl. For chipotle aioli, combine mayonnaise, lime juice, garlic, and chipotle pepper in a small bowl. Serve the shredded meat, the lettuce mixture, and the chipotle aioli in tortillas. Sprinkle with cilantro.

Tips: If desired, substitute ¼ teaspoon ground chipotle chile pepper for the canned chipotle pepper.

Leftover shredded meat can be stored in an airtight container in the refrigerator up to 3 days or freezer for up to 3 months.

Equipment: 3½- or 4-quart slow cooker

DAY 13

Tofu & Snow Pea Stir-Fry with Peanut Sauce

A fast dinner recipe perfect for busy weeknights, this easy stir-fry recipe will quickly become a favorite. To save time, use precooked rice or cook rice a day ahead.

Ingredients

4 servings

⅓ cup unsalted natural peanut butter3 tablespoons rice vinegar2 tablespoons low-sodium soy sauce2 teaspoons brown sugar (see Tip)2 teaspoons hot sauce, such as Sriracha1 (14 ounce) package extra-firm or firm tofu (see Tip)4 teaspoons canola oil, divided1 (14 ounce) package frozen (not thawed) pepper stir-fry vegetables2 tablespoons finely chopped or grated fresh ginger3 cloves garlic, minced2 cups fresh snow peas, trimmed2 tablespoons water, plus more if needed4 tablespoons unsalted roasted peanuts2 cups cooked brown rice

Preparation

Prep

30 m

Ready In

30 m

Combine peanut butter, vinegar, soy sauce, sugar, and hot sauce in a medium bowl; whisk until smooth. Set aside. Drain tofu; pat dry with a paper towel. Cut into ¾-inch cubes; pat dry again. Heat 2 tsp. oil in a large nonstick skillet over medium-high heat. Add half the tofu and let cook, undisturbed, until lightly browned underneath, about 2 minutes. Stir and continue cooking, stirring occasionally, until browned all over, 1 to 2 minutes. Transfer to a plate. Add 1 tsp. oil to the pan, then the remaining tofu; repeat. Add the remaining 1 tsp. oil to the pan. Add frozen vegetables, ginger, and garlic; stir-fry until the ginger and garlic are fragrant and the vegetables have thawed, 2 to 3 minutes. Stir in snow peas. Add water, cover and cook until the peas are crisp-tender, 3 to 4 minutes. Push the vegetables to the edges of the pan. Add the reserved peanut sauce to the center and cook, stirring, until hot, about 30 seconds. Stir the vegetables into the sauce. Add the reserved tofu and cook, stirring, until heated through, 30 to 60 seconds. If necessary, add more water to make a creamy sauce. Sprinkle each serving with 1 Tbsp. peanuts; serve with rice.

Tips: If using a sugar substitute, we recommend Splenda Brown Sugar Blend. Follow package directions for 2 tsp. equivalent. Nutrition Per Serving with Substitute: Same as below except CAL 506, CARB 47g (sugars 9g), POTASSIUM 316mg.

Don't like tofu? Substitute 12 oz. boneless, skinless chicken breast or chicken tenders, cut into thin slices. When you brown the chicken in Step 3, be sure that it is cooked through.

DAY 14

Chicken & Sun-Dried Tomato Orzo

Sun-dried tomatoes and Romano cheese pack a flavorful punch along with the tantalizing aroma of fresh marjoram in this rustic Italian-inspired dish. Serve with sautéed fresh spinach or steamed broccolini.

Ingredients 4 servings

8 ounces orzo, preferably whole-wheat1 cup water½ cup chopped sun-dried tomatoes, (not oil-packed), divided1 plum tomato, diced1 clove garlic, peeled3 teaspoons chopped fresh marjoram, divided1 tablespoon red-wine vinegar2 teaspoons plus 1 tablespoon extra-virgin olive oil, divided4 boneless, skinless chicken breasts, trimmed (1-1¼ pounds)¼ teaspoon salt¼ teaspoon freshly ground pepper1 9-ounce package frozen artichoke hearts, thawed½ cup finely shredded Romano cheese, divided

Preparation

Cook orzo in a large saucepan of boiling water until just tender, 8 to 10 minutes or according to package directions. Drain and rinse. Meanwhile, place 1 cup water, ¼ cup sun-dried tomatoes, plum tomato, garlic, 2 teaspoons marjoram, vinegar and 2 teaspoons oil in a blender. Blend until just a few chunks remain. Season chicken with salt and pepper on both sides. Heat remaining 1 tablespoon oil in a large skillet over medium-high heat. Add the chicken and cook, adjusting the heat as necessary to prevent burning, until golden outside and no longer pink in the middle, 3 to 5 minutes per side. Transfer to a plate; tent with foil to keep warm. Pour the tomato sauce into the pan and bring to a boil. Measure out ½ cup sauce to a small bowl. Add the remaining ¼ cup sun-dried tomatoes to the pan along with the orzo, artichoke hearts and 6 tablespoons cheese. Cook, stirring, until heated through, 1 to 2 minutes. Divide among 4 plates. Slice the chicken. Top each portion of pasta with sliced chicken, 2 tablespoons of the reserved tomato sauce and a sprinkling of the remaining cheese and marjoram.

DAY 15

Easy Pea & Spinach Carbonara

Fresh pasta cooks up faster than dried, making it a must-have for fast weeknight dinners like this luscious yet healthy meal. Eggs are the base of the creamy sauce. They don't get fully cooked, so use pasteurized-in-the-shell eggs if you prefer.

Ingredients

4 servings

1½ tablespoons extra-virgin olive oil½ cup panko breadcrumbs, preferably whole-wheat1 small clove garlic, minced8 tablespoons grated Parmesan cheese, divided3 tablespoons finely chopped fresh parsley3 large egg yolks1 large egg½ teaspoon ground pepper¼ teaspoon salt1 (9 ounce) package fresh tagliatelle or linguine8 cups baby spinach1 cup peas (fresh or frozen)

Preparation

Put 10 cups of water in a large pot and bring to a boil over high heat. Meanwhile, heat oil in a large skillet over medium-high heat. Add breadcrumbs and garlic; cook, stirring frequently, until toasted, about 2 minutes. Transfer to a small bowl and stir in 2 tablespoons Parmesan and parsley. Set aside. Whisk the remaining 6 tablespoons Parmesan, egg yolks, egg, pepper and salt in a medium bowl. Cook pasta in the boiling water, stirring occasionally, for 1 minute. Add spinach and peas and cook until the pasta is tender, about 1 minute more. Reserve ¼ cup of the cooking water. Drain and place in a large bowl. Slowly whisk the reserved cooking water into the egg mixture. Gradually add the mixture to the pasta, tossing with tongs to combine. Serve topped with the reserved breadcrumb mixture.

DAY 16

Hearty Tomato Soup with Beans & Greens

Garlicky kale and creamy white beans elevate simple canned tomato soup into a 10-minute lunch or dinner that really satisfies. Use a soup with tomato pieces for a heartier texture. Look for a brand that's low- or reduced-sodium, with no more than 450 mg sodium per serving

Ingredients

4 servings

2 (14 ounce) cans low-sodium hearty-style tomato soup1 tablespoon olive oil3 cups chopped kale1 teaspoon minced garlic⅛ teaspoon crushed red pepper (optional)1 (14 ounce) can no-salt-added cannellini beans, rinsed¼ cup grated Parmesan cheese

Preparation

Heat soup in a medium saucepan according to package directions; simmer over low heat as you prepare kale. Heat oil in a large skillet over medium heat. Add kale and cook, stirring, until wilted, 1 to 2 minutes. Stir in garlic and crushed red pepper (if using) and cook for 30 seconds. Stir the greens and beans into the soup and simmer until the beans are heated through, 2 to 3 minutes. Divide the soup among 4 bowls. Serve topped with Parmesan.

DAY 17

Curried Chickpea Stew

Who says a meatless meal isn't filling? Packed with fiber-rich vegetables and chickpeas, this fragrant stew satisfies.

Ingredients

8 servings

1 (10 ounce) bag prewashed spinach or other sturdy greens1½ tablespoons canola oil1 large onion, chopped1 (2 inch) piece fresh ginger, peeled and minced½-1 small jalapeño pepper, seeded and finely chopped3 cloves garlic, minced1 tablespoon curry powder3 medium carrots, peeled and thinly sliced½ medium head cauliflower, broken into bite-size florets (3 cups)2 (15 ounce) cans low-sodium chickpeas, rinsed2 (14 ounce) cans no-salt-added diced tomatoes, drained½ cup fat-free half-and-half⅓ cup "lite" coconut milk

Preparation

Place spinach (or other greens) in a microwave-safe dish; add 1 Tbsp. water and cover. Microwave on High, stirring occasionally, until just wilted, 1 to 2 minutes. Transfer to a colander to drain. When cool enough to handle, squeeze out any excess water. Coarsely chop and set aside. Heat oil in a large nonstick skillet with high sides or a Dutch oven. Add onion and cook, stirring, until translucent, about 8 minutes. Add ginger, jalapeño, garlic, and curry powder; cook, stirring, for 30 seconds. Add carrots and 2 Tbsp. water; cover and cook, stirring occasionally, until the carrots have softened, about 10 minutes (add more water if the mixture becomes dry). Add cauliflower; cover and cook, stirring occasionally, until barely tender-crisp, 5 to 10 minutes more. Stir in chickpeas, tomatoes, half-and-half, and coconut milk. Bring to just below boiling. Reduce heat to low and simmer uncovered, stirring occasionally, for 15 minutes. Stir in the reserved spinach (or greens) and heat through. Transfer half of the mixture (about 5 cups) to a 1½-qt. freezer container; label and freeze for up to 1 month. Serve the remaining half at once, or refrigerate for up to 3 days.

To make ahead: This double-batch recipe makes one meal for tonight (or to refrigerate for up to 3 days) and one to freeze for up to 1 month (see Step 4). To cook from frozen: Thaw overnight in the refrigerator, then microwave on High until heated through, 4 to 5 minutes. You can also reheat the stew in a saucepan until bubbling; add a little water, if needed, to prevent sticking.

DAY 18

Pork & Green Chile Stew

Let your slow cooker work—while you're at work!—and come home to a delicious bowl of hearty stew for dinner. Full of potatoes, hominy, green chiles, and chunks of pork sirloin, this filling stew recipe takes just 25 minutes to prepare in the morning.

Ingredients

6 servings

2 pounds boneless pork sirloin roast or shoulder roast1 tablespoon vegetable oil½ cup chopped onion (1 medium)4 cups peeled and cubed potatoes (4 medium)3 cups water1 (15 ounce) can hominy or whole-kernel corn, drained2 (4 ounce) cans diced green chile peppers, undrained2 tablespoons quick-cooking tapioca1 teaspoon garlic salt½ teaspoon ground cumin½ teaspoon ancho chile powder½ teaspoon ground pepper¼ teaspoon dried oregano, crushedChopped fresh cilantro (optional)

Preparation

Trim fat from meat. Cut the meat into ½-inch pieces. Cook half of the meat in a large skillet in hot oil over medium-high heat until browned. Using a slotted spoon, remove the meat from the skillet. Repeat with the remaining meat and the onion. Drain off fat. Transfer all of the meat and the onion to a 3½- to 4½-quart slow cooker. Stir in potatoes, the water, hominy, green chile peppers, tapioca, garlic salt, cumin, ancho chile powder, ground pepper, and oregano. Cover and cook on Low for 7 to 8 hours or on High for 4 to 5 hours. If desired, garnish each serving with cilantro.

Equipment: 3½- to 4½-quart slow cooker

DAY 19

Trapanese Pesto Pasta & Zoodles with Salmon

Trapanese pesto is the Sicilian version of the sauce that uses tomatoes and almonds instead of pine nuts. This savory pesto sauce coats low-carb zucchini noodles and heart-healthy seared salmon to create an absolutely delicious pasta dinner.

Ingredients

6 servings

2 zucchini (1¾ lbs. total)1 teaspoon salt, divided½ cup raw whole almonds, toasted1 pound grape tomatoes (3 cups)1 cup packed fresh basil leaves plus ¼ cup chopped, divided2-4 cloves garlic¼ teaspoon crushed red pepper3 tablespoons olive oil, divided8 ounces whole-wheat spaghetti1 pound skinless salmon fillets (about 4 fillets), patted dry¼ teaspoon ground pepper, plus more for garnish2 tablespoons grated Parmesan cheese (optional)

Preparation

Bring a large pot of water to a boil. Cut zucchini into long thin strips with a spiralizer or vegetable peeler. Place in a colander set over a large bowl. Toss with ¼ tsp. salt and let drain for 15 to 20 minutes. Meanwhile, pulse almonds in a food processor until coarsely chopped. Add tomatoes, 1 cup basil leaves, garlic, and crushed red pepper; pulse until coarsely chopped. Add 2 Tbsp. oil and ½ tsp. salt and pulse until combined; set aside. Cook spaghetti in the boiling water according to package directions. Drain and transfer to a large bowl. Gently squeeze the zucchini to remove excess water; add to the bowl with the spaghetti. Heat the remaining 1 Tbsp. oil in a large skillet over medium-high heat until shimmering. Season salmon with pepper and the remaining ¼ tsp. salt. Add the salmon to the pan; cook until the underside is golden and crispy, about 4 minutes. Flip the salmon and cook until it flakes when nudged with a fork, 2 to 4 minutes more. Transfer to a plate and use a fork to gently flake it apart. Add the pesto to the spaghetti mixture; toss to coat. Gently stir in the salmon. Top with the remaining ¼ cup chopped fresh basil. Garnish with Parmesan and additional pepper, if desired.

DAY 20

Jerk Chicken & Pineapple Slaw

Ready in under 30 minutes, this spicy chicken dish with sweet pinapple slaw is perfect for any night of the week.

Ingredients

4 servings

3 heads baby bok choy, trimmed and thinly sliced2 cups shredded red cabbage½ of a fresh pineapple, peeled, cored and chopped2 tablespoons cider vinegar4 teaspoons packed brown sugar2 teaspoons all-purpose flour2 teaspoons jerk seasoning4 skinless, boneless chicken breast halves (1 to 1¼ pounds total)

Preparation

For pineapple slaw, in a very large bowl combine bok choy, cabbage and pineapple. In a small bowl combine cider vinegar and 2 teaspoons of the brown sugar. Drizzle over bok choy mixture; toss to coat. Set aside. In a large resealable plastic bag combine the remaining 2 teaspoons brown sugar, the flour and jerk seasoning. Add chicken; shake well to coat. Grease a grill pan or a heavy 12-inch skillet. Add chicken;

cook over medium heat for 8 to 12 minutes or until no longer pink (170°F), turning once halfway through cooking time. Transfer chicken to a cutting board. Slice chicken and serve with pineapple slaw.

DAY 21

Jambalaya Stuffed Peppers

In this healthy stuffed peppers recipe, a delicious jambalaya filling of chicken and Cajun spices gets baked inside of bell peppers. Traditional jambalaya is made with green bell peppers, but you can use green, yellow, or orange peppers (or a mix) for this dish. Look for bell peppers with even bottoms, so that they stand upright on their own.

Ingredients

6 servings

6 large green, yellow, or orange bell peppers1½ pounds boneless, skinless chicken thighs, trimmed and cut into 1-inch pieces2 tablespoons salt-free Cajun seasoning (see Tip), divided2 tablespoons olive oil, divided1 link andouille sausage (3-4 oz.), sliced½ cup diced celery1 small onion, diced (½ cup)2 cloves garlic, minced½ teaspoon salt1 (14 ounce) can diced tomatoes¼ cup tomato paste1 cup low-sodium chicken broth1 cup uncooked instant brown rice

Preparation

Preheat oven to 400°F. Line a large rimmed baking sheet with parchment paper or foil. Cut tops off peppers and carefully remove the core and seeds, taking care not to split the skin. Dice the pepper tops and set aside. Place the peppers on the prepared baking sheet; bake for 20 minutes. Remove from oven and let cool. Discard any accumulated liquid in the bottom of the peppers. Meanwhile, season chicken on all sides with 1 Tbsp. Cajun seasoning. Heat 1 Tbsp. oil in a large skillet over medium heat. Add half of the chicken and cook, turning to brown all sides, 4 to 6 minutes. Transfer the chicken to a medium bowl with a slotted spoon. Repeat with the remaining 1 Tbsp. olive oil and the remaining chicken. Add sausage to the now-empty skillet and cook, stirring occasionally, until lightly browned, 1 to 2 minutes. Add celery, onion, and the reserved diced pepper; cook, stirring often, until the onions are translucent, 3 to 5 minutes. Add garlic, the remaining 1 Tbsp. Cajun seasoning, and salt; cook, stirring, for 30 seconds. Add tomatoes and tomato paste; stir to combine, scraping any brown bits off the bottom of the pan. Add broth, rice, and the chicken with any accumulated juices; stir to combine. Bring to a boil. Reduce heat to maintain a simmer and cook, stirring occasionally, until the chicken has cooked through and the rice has softened, 5 to 10 minutes. Remove from heat and stir. Let stand, covered, until all liquid is absorbed, about 10 minutes. Divide the chicken mixture among the peppers, spooning about 1¼ cups into each one and mounding it on top, if necessary. Bake until heated through, about 20 minutes.

Tip: We prefer homemade Cajun seasoning, because it has more flavor and fewer preservatives than the store-bought versions. For salt-free Cajun seasoning, mix 1 Tbsp. paprika, 1 tsp. each onion powder and garlic powder, ½ tsp. each dried oregano and thyme, and ¼ tsp. each cayenne and ground pepper. You will have slightly more than you need for this recipe; use it to season eggs, chicken, fish, or vegetables. (Want to have extra on hand? Multiply these amounts by four.) Store in a covered jar for up to 6 months.

OTHER MEALS ARE

Sweet Asian Beef Stir-Fry

This Asian-inspired beef stir-fry recipe is loaded with crisp-tender vegetables and served over spaghetti with a sweet orange-teriyaki sauce. If you don't have spaghetti noodles in your pantry, substitute soba noodles, rice or quinoa

Ingredients

4 servings

3 tablespoons low-sugar orange marmalade2 tablespoons light teriyaki sauce2 tablespoons water1 tablespoon grated fresh ginger¼ to ½ teaspoon crushed red pepper3 ounces dried multigrain spaghetti or soba (buckwheat) noodlesNonstick cooking spray2 cups small broccoli florets½ of a small red onion, cut into thin wedges1 cup packaged julienned carrots, or 2 carrots, cut into thin bite-size strips2 teaspoons canola oil12 ounces boneless beef top sirloin steak, cut into thin bite-size strips (see Tip)3 cups shredded napa cabbage

Preparation

In a small bowl, combine marmalade, teriyaki sauce, the water, ginger and crushed red pepper; set aside. Cook spaghetti according to package directions. Meanwhile, coat a large nonstick skillet or wok with cooking spray. Preheat over medium-high heat. Add broccoli and red onion to hot skillet. Cover and cook for 3 minutes, stirring occasionally. Add carrots; cover and cook for 3 to 4 minutes more or until vegetables are crisp-tender, stirring occasionally. Remove vegetables from skillet. Add oil to the same skillet. Add beef strips. Cook and stir over medium-high heat for 3 to 5 minutes or until slightly pink in center. Return vegetables to skillet along with sauce and cabbage. Cook and stir for 1 to 2 minutes or until heated through and cabbage is just wilted. Serve immediately over the hot cooked spaghetti.

Tip: For easier slicing, partially freeze the steak before cutting it.

Pork Skewers with Fruit Glaze

Here's a quick and easy entree for six—chunks of succulent pork loin and red and green bell peppers are threaded onto skewers and grilled with a sweet fruit glaze. Choose your favorite fruit preserve for the glaze, like apricot, red raspberry, or strawberry.

Ingredients

6 servings

1 egg, slightly beaten⅓ cup finely chopped water chestnuts¼ cup fine dry breadcrumbs2 teaspoons grated fresh ginger1 clove garlic, minced¼ teaspoon salt¼ teaspoon ground pepper1 pound lean ground pork loin1 large red, yellow, or green bell pepper, cut into 1-inch pieces⅔ cup desired flavor low-sugar fruit preserves¼ cup pineapple juice1 tablespoon lemon juice¼ teaspoon ground cardamom

Preparation

Prep

30 m

Ready In

40 m

Combine egg, water chestnuts, breadcrumbs, ginger, garlic, salt, and ground pepper in a large bowl. Add ground pork; mix well. Shape the pork mixture into 30 meatballs. Alternately thread the meatballs and bell pepper pieces on six long metal skewers, leaving ¼ inch between pieces; set aside. Prepare glaze: place fruit preserves in a small saucepan; snip any large pieces. Stir in pineapple juice, lemon juice, and cardamom. Bring to boiling; reduce heat. Simmer, uncovered, for 15 minutes. Set aside to cool for 10 minutes while the pork cooks (the glaze will thicken as it cools). For a charcoal grill, arrange medium-hot coals around a drip pan. Test for medium heat above the pan. Place the skewers on well greased grill rack over the pan. Cover; grill for 10 to 12 minutes or until the meatballs are no longer pink and the juices run clear. Brush with some of the fruit glaze. Immediately remove the skewers from the grill. (For a gas grill, preheat grill. Reduce heat to medium. Adjust for indirect cooking. Grill as above.) Serve the skewers with the remaining glaze.

Red Cabbage-Apple Cauliflower Gnocchi

Tender cabbage and a vibrant applesauce-mustard pan sauce are the perfect pairing for pillowy low-carb cauliflower gnocchi. Add diced chicken-apple sausage for extra protein.

Ingredients

4 servings

3 cups shredded red cabbage2 tablespoons water, divided1 tablespoon olive oil1 (12 ounce) bag frozen cauliflower gnocchi½ cup unsweetened applesauce1 tablespoon Dijon mustardFreshly ground pepper to taste

Preparation

Place cabbage in a large microwave-safe bowl or baking dish. Add 1 tablespoon water. Cover tightly and microwave on High until softened, about 5 minutes. Heat oil in a large skillet over medium-high heat. Add gnocchi and cook, stirring frequently, until browned, about 5 minutes. Add cabbage and the remaining 1 tablespoon water; cover and cook, stirring occasionally, until the water evaporates. Stir in applesauce and mustard and heat through. Season with pepper.

Chicken-Spaghetti Squash Bake

In this version of a chicken-and-broccoli casserole, spaghetti squash takes on a creamy texture when baked with cream of mushroom soup.

Ingredients

8 servings

1 medium spaghetti squash (about 3 lbs.)4 cups broccoli florets1 tablespoon canola oil1 (10 ounce) package sliced mushrooms1 medium onion, finely chopped2 cloves garlic, minced½ teaspoon dried thyme½ teaspoon ground pepper2 (10 ounce) cans reduced-sodium condensed cream of mushroom soup, such as Campbell's 25% Less Sodium1½ pounds boneless, skinless chicken breasts, cut into bite-size pieces½ cup shredded extra-sharp Cheddar cheese

Preparation

Prep

55 m

Ready In

1 h 40 m

Preheat oven to 375°F. Coat two 8-inch-square baking dishes with cooking spray. Halve squash lengthwise and scoop out the seeds. Place cut-side down in a microwave-safe dish; add 2 Tbsp. water. Microwave, uncovered, on High until the flesh can be scraped with a fork but is still tender-crisp, 10 to 12 minutes. Scrape the strands onto a plate; set aside. Place broccoli in the same microwave-safe dish; add 1 Tbsp. water and cover. Microwave on High, stirring occasionally, until just barely tender-crisp, 2 to 3 minutes. Drain and set aside to cool. Meanwhile, heat oil in a large nonstick skillet over medium-high heat. Add mushrooms and cook, stirring, until they've released their juices, about 8 minutes. Add onion and continue cooking until the onion is tender and the mushrooms are lightly browned, about 8 minutes. Stir in garlic, thyme, and pepper; cook, stirring, for 30 seconds, Stir in soup (do not dilute with water) and heat through. Stir in chicken and the reserved squash and broccoli; gently toss to combine well. Divide the mixture between the prepared baking dishes and sprinkle each with ¼ cup Cheddar. Cover with foil. Label and freeze one casserole for up to 1 month.

Bake the remaining casserole until bubbling, about 25 minutes. Uncover and continue baking until lightly browned along the edges, 10 to 15 minutes more. Let stand for 10 minutes before serving.

To make ahead: This double-batch recipe makes one casserole for tonight and one to freeze for up to 1 month (see Step 6). To cook from frozen: Thaw overnight in the refrigerator. Spoon off any liquid that has accumulated in the pan, if desired. Bake as directed in Step 7.

Equipment: Two 8-inch-square baking dishes or foil pans

Loaded Black Bean Nacho Soup

Jazz up a can of black bean soup with your favorite nacho toppings, such as cheese, avocado and fresh tomatoes. A bit of smoked paprika adds a bold flavor kick, but you can swap in any warm spices you prefer, such as cumin or chili powder. Look for a soup that contains no more than 450 mg sodium per serving.

Ingredients

2 servings

1 (18 ounce) carton low-sodium black bean soup¼ teaspoon smoked paprika½ teaspoon lime juice½ cup halved grape tomatoes½ cup shredded cabbage or slaw mix2 tablespoons crumbled cotija cheese or other Mexican-style shredded cheese½ medium avocado, diced2 ounces baked tortilla chips

Preparation

Pour soup into a small saucepan and stir in paprika. Heat according to package directions. Stir in lime juice. Divide the soup between 2 bowls and top with tomatoes, cabbage (or slaw), cheese and avocado. Serve with tortilla chips.

Pesto Shrimp Pasta

Using a packaged pesto sauce mix saves time in this 20-minute orzo pasta salad recipe.

Ingredients

4 servings

1 cup dried orzo (6 ounces)4 teaspoons packaged pesto sauce mix, such as Knorr brand, divided2 tablespoons olive oil, divided1 pound peeled and deveined fresh or frozen medium shrimp, thawed1 medium zucchini, halved lengthwise and

sliced⅛ teaspoon coarse salt⅛ teaspoon freshly cracked pepper1 lemon, halved1 ounce shaved Parmesan cheese

Preparation

Prepare orzo pasta according to package directions. Drain; reserving ¼ cup of the pasta cooking water. Stir 1 teaspoon of the pesto mix into the reserved cooking water; set aside. While pasta is boiling, combine 3 teaspoons of the pesto mix and 1 tablespoon of the olive oil in a large resealable plastic bag. Seal and shake to combine. Add shrimp to bag; seal and turn to coat. Set aside. Cook zucchini in a large skillet in the remaining 1 tablespoon hot oil over medium-high heat for 1 to 2 minutes, stirring often. Add the pesto-marinated shrimp to the skillet and cook for 4 to 5 minutes or until shrimp is opaque. Add the cooked pasta to the skillet with the zucchini and shrimp mixture. Stir in the reserved pasta water until absorbed, scraping up any seasoning in the bottom of the pan. Season with salt and pepper. Squeeze the lemon halves over the pasta just before serving. Top with Parmesan.

Honey Mustard Salmon with Mango Quinoa

In this 30-minute dinner recipe, grilled, honey mustard-coated salmon is served with a tasty grain salad made with quinoa, mango, jalapeño and almonds.

Ingredients

2 servings

1 (8 ounce) fresh or frozen skinless salmon fillet2 teaspoons honey2 teaspoons spicy brown mustard1 large clove garlic, minced⅔ cup cooked quinoa, room temperature½ cup chopped fresh or frozen mango, thawed if frozen1 to 2 tablespoons seeded and finely chopped fresh jalapeño chile pepper (see Tip)1 tablespoon sliced almonds, toasted (see Tip)1 teaspoon olive oil⅛ teaspoon saltPinch ground black pepper2 tablespoons chopped fresh cilantro

Preparation

Thaw salmon, if frozen. Rinse fish and pat dry with paper towels. In a small bowl, stir together honey, mustard and garlic. Brush both sides of salmon with honey mixture. For a gas or charcoal grill, place salmon on grill rack directly over medium heat. Cover and grill for 4 to 6 minutes per ½-inch thickness of fish until salmon begins to flake when tested with a fork, turning once. Meanwhile, in a medium bowl, stir together quinoa, mango, jalapeño pepper, almonds, olive oil, salt and black pepper. Top with fresh cilantro. Serve salmon with quinoa.

Tips: Because chile peppers contain volatile oils that can burn your skin and eyes, avoid direct contact with them as much as possible. When working with chile peppers, wear plastic or rubber gloves. If your bare hands do touch the peppers, wash your hands and nails well with soap and warm water.

To toast nuts, spread in a shallow baking pan lined with parchment paper. Bake in a 350°F oven for 5 to 10 minutes or until golden, shaking pan once or twice.

Pork Tenderloin with Apple-Onion Chutney

If you'd like the chutney in this pork tenderloin recipe to be both sweet and tart, opt for sweet apples like red or golden delicious and sweet onion.

Ingredients

2 servings

1 (8 ounce) piece pork tenderloin⅛ teaspoon dried thyme, crushed⅛- ¼ teaspoon pepper¾ cup thinly sliced onion8 ounces apples, cored and sliced¼ cup water2 tablespoons

cider vinegar1 teaspoon honey¼ teaspoon salt⅛ teaspoon ground cumin (optional)Chopped fresh thyme (optional)

Preparation

Trim fat from pork. Cut the meat in half crosswise. Place each piece, cut side down, between two pieces of plastic wrap. Working from center to edges, pound lightly with the flat side of a meat mallet to ½-inch thickness. Remove the plastic wrap. Sprinkle the meat with dried thyme and pepper. Lightly coat an unheated large skillet with cooking spray. Add the pork. Cook over medium-high heat for 6 to 9 minutes or until a thermometer inserted in the pork registers 145°F, turning once halfway through cooking. Transfer the pork to a plate. Cover and keep warm. For chutney, cook onion in the same skillet about 4 minutes or until tender, stirring occasionally. Stir in apple slices, the water, vinegar, honey, salt, and cumin (if desired). Bring to boiling; reduce heat. Simmer, uncovered, for 4 to 5 minutes or until the liquid is almost evaporated and the apples are tender, stirring occasionally. Return the pork to the skillet and heat through. Divide the pork and chutney between two plates. If desired, garnish with fresh thyme.

Do not go yet; One last thing to do

If you enjoyed this book or found it useful I'd be very grateful if you'd post a short review on it. Your support really does make a difference and I read all the reviews personally so I can get your feedback and make this book even better.

Thanks again for your support!